D0463601

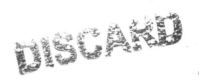

TAKING LIBERTIES

TAKING LIBERTIES

EDITED BY

ERICA CARTER & SIMON WATNEY

SERPENT'S
TAIL

Published in association with the ICA

British Library Cataloguing in Publication Data

Taking Liberties: AIDS and cultural politics.
1. Man. AIDS. Social aspects
I. Carter, Erica. II. Watney, Simon
362.1'042

ISBN 1-85242-147-9

First published in 1989 by
Serpent's Tail, 4 Blackstock Mews, London N4

Typeset in 10/12 pt Garamond by
AKM Associates (UK) Ltd., Southall, London

Printed in Great Britain by
WBC Print (Bristol) Ltd.

CONTENTS

TAKING LIBERTIES

PREFACE

Taking Liberties emerges out of a conference at the Institute of Contemporary Arts (ICA), London, on 5 and 6 March 1988. Our hope for the book is that it will rekindle discussions begun in the '88 conference. Some of the articles published here are closely based on conference papers, others have been substantially elaborated, and yet others separately commissioned from conference participants — audience and speakers.

The concerns voiced in *Taking Liberties* represent a broad diversity of cultural, political and ethical issues; its contributors speak from a variety of perspectives — as journalists, community activists, academics and public sector workers. What unites their work is a common understanding of AIDS as fundamentally challenging the meanings, values and practices in which our experiences of sexuality, love, the body, life, death and physical processes are grounded. A common impulse is discernible in contributions to *Taking Liberties*: the desire to set an agenda for debate and action on AIDS outside the professional arenas of science, medicine and social welfare — the insistence that AIDS has reverberations across the whole spectrum of cultural practices, and that strategies against it must *always* take account of AIDS in its cultural dimension.

These strategies are elaborated from diverse standpoints within the book. A number of authors address issues of representation: representation as depiction in text and image — Judith Williamson on genre, Simon Watney on language, AIDS and the third world, Jan Zita Grover on metaphor — or in its more conventionally political sense, as participation in the democratic process; thus Keith Alcorn looks at the questions AIDS poses for public service broadcasting as a vehicle for the formation of a democratic public sphere; Erica Carter examines the place of the "committed" intellectual in AIDS activism, while Richard Goldstein addresses the notion of a renewed social contract as a platform from which the epidemic can be most successfully combated. Many contributors — Lynne Segal, for example, who argues forcefully for a pro-sex, feminist politics of AIDS — turn their attention to questions of sexual rights and freedoms, and strategies against the moral backlash which AIDS is used to legitimate. Running through *Taking Liberties* is, too, a recurrent concern with the politics of health and the body in both the personal and the public political arena. Cindy Patton, Jeffrey Weeks, Tom Stoddard and Tony Whitehead address the delicate balance between community mobilization and the professionalization of AIDS work nationally and internationally; Meurig Horton examines placebo drug trials in the context of a repressive history of medical discourse; and in his introduction, Simon Watney sketches out the implications of the book for a cultural politics of AIDS in late eighties' Britain.

This is a collection that insists on the necessary diversity of responses to AIDS. While some contributors, notably Jonathan Grimshaw and Michael Bronski, give accounts of individual experiences of HIV infection and its emotional consequences, others focus on the common issues faced by different communities in their encounters with AIDS — questions of sexual repressions and freedoms, of access to knowledge and information, of social stigma, sexism and classism, political irresponsibility.

For their support in that endeavour, we owe thanks to individuals and groups too numerous to mention. We would like however to acknowledge a particular debt of gratitude to the following: the ICA and its restaurant, Work in Progress, who provided the back-up needed to stage the conference, and whose staff supported us enthusiastically throughout the project. We would also like to take this opportunity to thank Craig Owens for his enthusiastic support in the early stages of planning the conference. In the event he was sadly unable to get to London; his "absence" was felt as a keen "presence". Thanks in particular to Katy Sender, Debbie Woolf and Andrea Lazar, and to Andrew Baggett and Julia Malandine for help with typing. We also wish to thank the Health Education Authority, and in particular Mukesh Kapila and Derek Bodell for their continued encouragement. Finally, thanks to Pete Ayrton and John Hampson of Serpent's Tail, for sustained support and judicious memory-jogging when deadlines threatened . . .

EC/SW, September 1988–March 1989

discussed in detail include the systematic denial of insurance, housing, welfare benefits, and basic health care provision, especially in the form of treatment drugs, to people with HIV infection or related disease. The racial and sexual political dimensions of the epidemic were also tackled, in front of a huge audience. At the end of a long and exhausting day, New York City's commissioner of health, Dr Stephen Joseph, stood up to repeat the familiar litany of tired and lame excuses for City Hall's shocking record of neglect in all areas of AIDS related funding, policy and practice. In the meantime however, Kramer and others were marching up and down in front of the speakers' podium with large placards, like subtitles to a foreign language film, announcing: "This Man's Lying", "Would You Believe This Man?", and simply, "Murderer".

This all speaks of a level of public involvement and engagement which remains sadly absent in the United Kingdom, where AIDS has not yet been widely taken up as a political or cultural issue, in spite of the fact that the situation of people with AIDS here is in many ways as bad as in the United States, where the Constitution and Bill of Rights at least provide some protection against a climate of appalling injustice. The difference between our two national responses to the epidemic was clearly evident in the early months of 1987 by the formation in New York of the AIDS Coalition To Unleash Power (ACT UP)[3]. An open invitation was distributed around the *Village Voice* Teach-In by ACT UP secretary Bradley Ball: "Over twenty thousand American men, women and children of all colours, gay and straight, have died of AIDS. The Centers for Disease Control project that another one and a half million are infected; the World Health Organization estimates that in five to ten years, one hundred million people globally will be infected or have the syndrome. As New York City residents, we are living in the AIDS capital of the nation, with over one third of all reported cases. Seven years into this epidemic, the National Institute of Health is *still* not testing many promising drugs for people with AIDS; the Food and Drug Administration is *still* not releasing the few drugs that have been tested; Mayor Koch *still* treats the crisis as if it were an outbreak of measles; the Department of Health and Human Services continues to ignore the recommendations of its own Surgeon General, Dr C. Everett Koop; and the Reagan administration has failed to establish a co-ordinated comprehensive national policy of AIDS. Outraged by this gross negligence, a diverse non-partisan group of individuals has united to form the AIDS Coalition To Unleash Power (ACT UP). Our goal is to demonstrate our anger and frustration at this intolerable situation, create a critical mass of informed public opinion, and influence our leaders to take constructive action. We need your support. We encourage you to join us at out weekly meetings and to participate in our demonstrations . . . We must fight together to overcome this tragedy."

These words are equally relevant to the situation in Britain today, where more than a thousand people have already died from AIDS; where the private pharmaceutical industry dominates such few treatment research projects as are underway; where patient care is extremely uneven; where treatment drugs are frequently unavailable; where life insurance and job and work security are systematically denied to all those perceived as at risk for HIV according to *demographic* factors rather than relevant risk factors such as whether people practice Safer Sex; where the mass media continues to pump out social and medical misinformation which puts increasing numbers of people at *real* risk of infection; where public health education has still totally failed to address the communities most devastated by AIDS; where the vilification of people with HIV and AIDS is more extreme than anywhere else in the western world; and where Health Minister David Mellor recently followed up the observation that as many as one in four gay men in London may have been infected — on this estimate perhaps a quarter of a million —with the comment that: "People must not breathe a sigh of relief and think it will soon blow over."[4] I hope I do not have to enlarge on the truly terrifying implications of that statement. Suffice to say that it is tragically clear that large sections of the population of Britain are not officially regarded as "people" at all.

In 1986, I approached the Institute of Contemporary Arts, in London, with a proposal for a conference which might consider British and American responses to AIDS, with invited speakers from both countries. No funding was forthcoming at that time, despite extensive efforts and enquiries on the part of Erica Carter and Katy Sender from the ICA. Indeed, the conference that eventually took place in March of 1988, and of which this book is in part a record, only took place at all as a result of direct support from the Health Education Authority, which underwrote the cost of admission for all AIDS workers in both the voluntary and statutory sectors. Whilst the conference was, I think, a great success, and well attended, the familiar ICA audience of feminists, academics, leftists, cultural workers, critics and theorists, was in the main conspicuous only by its absence. I have no reason to believe that the situation would be significantly different today. In spite of the long tradition of cultural studies in Britain, and endless discussion of the so-called "new social movements", it seems that lesbians and gay men are still very much on our own in the present crisis, and that the groups and political movements that we have energetically supported over the past two decades are not yet willing or able to recognize or respond to the political dimension of AIDS in Britain. Pious words are frequently heard concerning the "tragedy" of AIDS in the conveniently far-away developing world. But for those denied adequate medical care, and the most basic social welfare provision in the UK, there are as yet few advocates or allies. The attention of the left and middle ground of British culture and politics has not so far been directed towards the AIDS crisis in Britain, and one of the several aims of this book is to establish such vital connections, and the relations between the epidemic and other areas of contemporary cultural politics.

AIDS or HIV Disease?

In 1981 doctors in New York and Los Angeles independently reported significant clusters of two previously rare medical conditions — pneumocystis carinii pneumonia (PCP) and a form of cancer known as Kaposi's sarcoma (KS).[5] The only connection between these and a number of other rare diseases shortly reported amongst otherwise healthy young gay men, was their known association with damage to the body's immunological defences. Because these clusters were first identified among gay men, they were collectively described as Gay Related Immune Deficiency (GRID). It was eventually recognized (and not without considerable resistance on the part of some doctors and epidemiologists) that the underlying cause was not specific to gay men as such, especially after the discovery that the unknown agent underlying the various symptoms could be transmitted via blood transfusions. Thus, in 1982, the Centers for Disease Control (CDC) in Atlanta, Georgia, officially classified the resulting conditions as Acquired Immune Deficiency Syndrome (AIDS), by which name they are still widely known.

The Human Immunodeficiency Virus (HIV), which is responsible for AIDS, was not isolated until 1983, and not made public until the following year. In all of this it is most important to recognize that doctors, and members of the gay community, were working *backwards*, in a detective manner, in order to establish the agent or agents responsible for the syndrome of conditions categorized collectively as AIDS, and to understand its possible modes of transmission, in order to protect people. Thus it was that Michael Callen and Richard Berkowitz wrote their ground-breaking pamphlet "How To Have Sex In An Epidemic", with a preface by Dr Joseph Sonnabend, in New York in 1983, on the assumption that a sexually transmissable agent, or agents, was responsible for many if not all cases of AIDS. This was the originating moment of what we all now know as Safer Sex, and it pre-dated the isolation of HIV. None the less, even now, the distinction between HIV and AIDS is far from universally understood, and AIDS is widely regarded as if it were a single *disease*, rather than a *syndrome*, comprising a large number of distinct diseases, tumours, cancers, and so on, which may occur in many different combinations and sequences in the wake of HIV infection and damage to the body's immunological defences.

Hence the need to emphasize that AIDS is not a single condition, and that different people with AIDS do not necessarily share medical or clinical experience. It is not widely known that people with AIDS, on average, spend less than 20 per cent of their lives after diagnosis in hospital. Nor is it appreciated that there is an average of eight years between initial HIV infection and the onset of classifiable AIDS symptoms, though this average is not *predictive* for any particular individual. We simply do not know how many people with HIV will eventually develop AIDS, or whether AIDS is invariably fatal. As Sir Thomas Browne pointed out in the early seventeenth century: "It is the heaviest stone that melancholy can throw at a man, to tell him he is at the end of his nature."[6] Having lived with AIDS for seven years, Michael Callen eloquently insists that the uncritical assertion that everyone with AIDS will die as a direct result of the syndrome "denies the reality of — but perhaps more important, the possibility of —our survival".[7] The use of treatment drugs that can retard the replication of HIV, strengthen the body's immunological defences, and prevent individual AIDS conditions, have already greatly increased the average life expectancy of previously healthy people with AIDS in the United States — at least those who are fortunate enough to have medical insurance, or who can get onto experimental drug trials.

It is this kind of straightforward information which is often difficult to communicate because of the way in which AIDS was first classified in 1982. Many of the most basic misunderstandings about HIV infection and AIDS stem from a fundamental failure by journalists and others who mediate medical information to non-professionals, to appreciate the significance of the distinction between HIV, with its well-established, limited modes of transmission, and AIDS. To describe the syndrome as if it were a disease is an easy option, but it obscures almost all the real issues faced by people with AIDS, and has led to any number of misleading assumptions and ill-informed beliefs about almost every aspect of the epidemic. For example, many people still talk about "catching AIDS", as if you could contract a syndrome. Repeated references to the so-called "AIDS virus" and "AIDS carriers" also remain a powerful barrier to effective health education, only serving to encourage the equally unfortunate belief that there is an "AIDS test" — as if a single blood test could possibly be sensitive to, or predict, the possible onset of all the various conditions categorized as AIDS, as well as the presence or absence of HIV.

There are thus strong reasons why we should consider following the example of the many doctors and health educators who have by-passed the category of AIDS, just as AIDS was used to by-pass the earlier classification of GRID. They talk of HIV infection, referring to the specific and clearly recognized modes of transmission of the virus; and HIV disease, referring to the progressive immuno-suppression that may follow in the wake of infection, making the body vulnerable to individual so-called "opportunistic" conditions such as KS and PCP. There is also another compelling reason why we should consider this a significant advance. As knowledge concerning the effects of HIV grew in the mid 1980s, it became clear that a large number of infected people were becoming seriously —and sometimes fatally — ill, though they did not have illnesses that are officially classified as AIDS. The revision and enlargement of the diagnostic category of AIDS by the CDC in August 1987 has still not improved the situation of all those people who find themselves diagnosed as people with AIDS Related Complex (ARC), sometimes known as AIDS Related Conditions. A diagnosis of ARC is in some ways even more difficult for many patients, than a diagnosis of either HIV or AIDS, since it is perceived as a "half-way house", nebulous yet only too real, an anxiety-inducing antechamber to the eventual emergence of AIDS. This only serves to encourage the use of absurd terms like "full-blown AIDS", to refer to people with any of the forty or more distinct conditions which collectively constitute the syndrome, as if people with ARC have "half" or "semi-blown" AIDS! Such commentary also obscures the wide range of experience of ARC and AIDS, from great pain and debilitation, to feelings of relative or complete good health.

It should be apparent that nobody deliberately set out to construct this Chinese box of bewildering medical categories, with all the confusion which they reinforce. The most practical and helpful solution would be to abandon gradually the categories of ARC and AIDS altogether, and to encourage the adoption of the simpler — and more accurate — distinction between HIV infection and HIV disease. In this way many thousands of people would be spared the unnecessary stress of an ARC diagnosis, which is a cruel and sadistic category with which nobody should be obliged to identify their experience of HIV disease and its many subsequences. This would have the added advantage of undermining much of the demonizing mythology surrounding the entire subject of AIDS. It would also make the task of health education much easier, and by making the epidemic more readily comprehensible, might help in the crucial task of preventing new cases of HIV infection. This is a particularly urgent priority, since the British government's AIDS education campaigns have consistently and conspicuously refused to clarify the distinction between HIV and AIDS, or to challenge the authority of mass media coverage of the epidemic — coverage which, it must be emphasized, only threatens to put newspaper readers and TV viewers at *increased* risk of HIV infection, by routinely providing ambiguous, misleading and conflicting messages.

AIDS Information as Ideological Practice
Whilst it is sometimes tempting to qualify attitudes towards HIV as "ignorant", or based on "misunderstanding", this ignores the more important point that public AIDS information has successfully established a widespread "knowledge" of the epidemic. This "knowledge" is perhaps most readily apparent in the closely related forms of questionnaires and opinion polls. Thus readers of the *Chicago Tribune* were recently asked whether it is true or false that "You can get AIDS from a water fountain," whether "A person can't

become infected with the AIDS virus by injecting drugs only once or twice," and so on.[8]

Through all of this, and countless other examples, the assumption runs that AIDS is indeed a disease, a unitary phenomenon which can be "caught". In the visual register we are repeatedly shown the faces and bodies of "AIDS victims" easily identified by the visible symptoms of KS, or by extremes of physical debilitation. AIDS is always the central term in such commentary, taking into itself the question of HIV transmission, and endlessly re-enacting the historical sequence which established AIDS as the central term through which the epidemic is conceived, to the virtual exclusion of the subsequently identified HIV. Yet AIDS educators working in the voluntary sector have met nothing but resistance on the part of journalists, doctors, and many professional health educators, to our insistence that effective health promotion requires a clearly established distinction between HIV and the Acquired Immune Deficiency Syndrome. Indeed, it sometimes feels as if there are two epidemics: one being described by the press and government agencies, the other being lived and resisted in the communities most directly affected by the effects of HIV infection and disease.

We will only fully understand the dramatic differences of emphasis and strategy between the voluntary and statutory sectors' responses to AIDS in terms of an analysis which recognizes the ways in which "official" AIDS information participates actively in the ideological foreground of all Western societies, seemingly validating social values and boundaries with the full authority of "science", and excluding whole population groups from what Stuart Hall has described as "the imaginary community of the nation".[9] At the same time, the supposed defence of "the nation" is ever more stridently invoked in order to justify measures that do nothing to help people with HIV, or to help prevent its transmission. In the meantime "the nation" is defined ever more sharply as the basic category with which good "healthy" citizens should identify.

Today's AIDS statistics reflect transmission events that took place, on average, some eight years ago, at a time when the very existence of HIV was completely unknown and unsuspected. It is therefore hardly surprising that the virus was widely transmitted in the two social constituencies that were seemingly affected first in the West — injecting drug users, and gay men. Although in the overall British and United States' epidemics the latter constitute the great majority of cases, there are always significant regional variations. For example, the majority of cases in Edinburgh are amongst injecting drug users and their sexual partners; this is also the overall picture in several European countries taken as a whole, including Italy and Spain. Hence the significance of Jan Zita Grover's argument elsewhere in this book that wherever possible we should think of AIDS on a local scale. Whilst it is of course convenient to generalize in comparisons between Britain and the United States, we should note that both countries are in fact experiencing a complex sequence of unfolding and overlapping epidemics, affecting different population groups, relative to different modes of transmission, and differing degress of access to health education, clean needles, drug treatments, and general standards of health care and social service provision. Wherever we look in the world, it is invariably the case that people's experience of HIV infection and disease faithfully duplicates their social and economic situation *before* the epidemic began.

HIV has had an overwhelming disproportionate initial effect on the marginal and the disadvantaged. In the early years of the epidemic so much attention was paid to the social groups that were affected first, that it was widely presented as if it were somehow a result of simply being black, or poor, or gay, or an injecting drug user forced to share needles. The widespread resistance to acknowledging the long-established fact of heterosexual transmission is not simply an example of "ignorance" or "misinformation": it stems directly from the ideological construction of AIDS as emblematic of otherness. Indeed, the complex history of AIDS-related legislation and official AIDS publicity demonstrates time and time again that the epidemic has been used to articulate values and beliefs that have nothing to do with AIDS. In effect, health education has been recruited to the prior purposes of political and ideological struggle. For such purposes it has seemed far more important to establish the idea that homosexuality is an intrinsic wrong, than to communicate the relatively simple information that explains how and why different people are at different degrees of risk from HIV.

The language of epidemiology has proved particularly useful in this respect. For example, gay men may technically be described as a "high-risk group" to the extent that we were affected early on in the history of the epidemic, long before HIV was known to exist. Yet instead of being understood as a group at high risk of contracting

HIV, gay men are widely regarded as constituting a high risk to other people. All around the world, from India to the United States, immigration requirements for HIV antibody testing speak volumes about the symbolic dimension of public AIDS commentary, and the social policies that it encourages. In this context we may distinguish between two basic approaches to AIDS education, which I have described elsewhere as the Terrorist Model and the Missionary Model.[10] For the former approach, HIV is regarded as an external invader, an illegal immigrant shinning up the white cliffs of Dover, a dangerous alien subversive slipping into the country unnoticed through Heathrow or JFK Airport, an enemy submarine sliding invisibly underwater up the belly of a fjord. From this perspective people with HIV are "AIDS carriers", and the distinction between HIV infection and disease is further obscured in the picture of a simple technological "solution" to the perceived problem — the so-called "AIDS test". The Terrorist Model therefore prescribes HIV testing, with varying degrees of compulsion, based on the fantasy that everyone with HIV can be detected, and the epidemic thereby halted. HIV testing is thus regarded as a means of primary prevention, rather than as a means of access to health care provision, and is justified on behalf of an imagined uninfected "general public", with little or no concern for infected individuals. It is axiomatic to this position that AIDS is regarded as a unitary disease, with no significant variations of symptoms or of life-expectancy, and no mention whatsoever of effective treatment interventions. It is in this grim light that quarantine or other punitive measures are frequently recommended. HIV is not seen as a problem for those infected; on the contrary, they are seen as a problem for "society", from membership of which they are immediately removed by their diagnosis.

For the Missionary Model, HIV is essentially understood as a kind of evil spirit, taking possession of its "victims". It appears as a heathen entity, strange and exotic —thriving on immorality, bestiality, unnatural acts and ungodly practices, of which it is also seen as a product. The "solution" from this perspective is therefore sought in a return to the supposedly "traditional" values of Judaeo-Christian morality, and its attendant institutions, above all marriage and "the family". Health education is replaced by notions of conversion, with a wedding ring offered as the most secure form of prophylaxis. Indeed, AIDS is often depicted from this point of view as if it were a spontaneously generated symptom of the divorce rates, always described as "soaring", and general levels of so-called "permissiveness". Chastity or monogamous heterosexual marriage are thus invoked as the only sure form of protection against an enemy presented as the insidious viral embodiment of a larger catastrophic breakdown of divine order. It is however important to note that this approach is not necessarily couched in such frankly religious terms, since it is equally characteristic of the national response to AIDS in many "socialist" countries, including Cuba and the Soviet Union. Yet whatever form its public rhetoric assumes, the Missionary Model presents the epidemic as symptomatic of a breakdown of moral hierarchies, order and authority, thus requiring a primarily moral solution, in order to "save" the Holy or the Pure. In this picture of things, people with HIV are clearly understood to be personally responsible and to blame for their condition, either as "sinners" or as "deviants", and their appearance has to closely reflect the enormity of their criminal depravity. Again, there is no question of treatment for such miscreants, beyond the administration of charity. Once AIDS is read as evidence of divine retribution or natural justice, the question of therapeutic treatment for people with HIV is all but unthinkable. To cure would seem to condone. "They've brought it on themselves," the logic runs, "and must suffer the inevitable consequences." From this perspective, having HIV is a juridical diagnosis, clearly understood as a capital offence.

Aspects of both the Terrorist and the Missionary models are generally to be found wherever AIDS publicity has been formally developed, with one usually predominant. The former tends to be more characteristic of Western social democracies, including the USA, whilst the latter is more characteristic of government policies and attitudes in the developing world. Yet both models are able to draw on local cultural and ideological formations in ways that are idiosyncratic and unpredictable. Actual policies thus tend towards compromise between conflicting imperatives, or, as in Britain and the USA, towards starkly contradictory and conflicting measures. Thus in Britain for example, the government's AIDS education programme has reflected a low-profile anti-interventionist neo-liberal school of thought, rather than the aggressive moralism of its neo-conservative wing. Yet at the same time the Department of Health and the Department of Education and Science have felt sufficiently confident to step in to censor education materials produced by the government's own Health Education Authority on the grounds that they do not sufficiently toe the "correct" moral Missionary line.[11] Nor should we forget that on the very day the Thatcher government was signing the declaration against AIDS-related discrimination which concluded the Global AIDS Summit in London, Clause 28 of the Local Government Bill (1987) was being enthusiastically endorsed across the road in the House of Commons.[12] The eventual wording of what passed into law as Section 28 of the Local Government Act of 1988, embodies a series of profoundly significant ideological motifs. These explain many of the contradictions and the glaring absences that have been so typical of the British government's responses to the epidemic.

Section 28 states that:
(1) A local authority shall not:
   (a) intentionally promote homosexuality or publish material with the intention of promoting homosexuality;
   (b) promote the teaching in any maintained school of the acceptability of homosexuality as a pretended family relationship.

(2) Nothing in subsection (1) above shall be taken to prohibit the doing of anything for the purpose of treating or preventing the spread of disease.

In order to understand the extraordinarily complex and difficult situation in which community-based AIDS educators find themselves, it is necessary to unpick some of the ideological threads that hold together this powerful and now legally binding view of the world. There are four key concepts which are closely locked together here: homosexuality, the family, teaching and disease. Stepping back a little from the actual wording of the legislation we can see that there is a central distinction between "pretended" and, by implication, "real" families. The law aims to prevent lesbian or gay relationships from being represented as if they are "real" family relationships. Furthermore, it is implied that any family with openly lesbian or gay members is somehow "unreal". Stepping back still further we can see that homosexuality is identified as a threat, to the extent that its "promotion" could undermine "real" families, either by actively seducing heterosexuals into homosexuality, or more simply by challenging the absolute supremacy of marriage as the only legitimate institution validating adult sexual relationships. From this point of view, lesbian and gay relationships are not only illegitimate, they are "unreal".

Section 28 is, of course, obliged to acknowledge that homosexuality exists, but can only explain its existence in terms of a crude conspiracy theory which regards lesbians and gay man as sinister predatory seducers, eagerly "promoting" our perversions to the young and "innocent". It thus speaks from a long tradition of legal moralism, dedicated to the protection of the supposedly "vulnerable".[13] Significantly, there is no attempt to legislate against specific sexual acts. On the contrary, Section 28 tacitly recognizes that the two decades prior to the emergence of HIV have been characterized by what Jeffrey Weeks has described as: "a decisive move away from the morality of 'acts' which had dominated sexual theorizing for hundreds of years and in the direction of a new relational perspective which takes into account context and meaning."[14] It is the field of lesbian and gay *culture* that Section 28 targets, where our personal and collective identities and political confidence are formed and validated. As the Prime Minister insisted at the 1987 Tory Party conference: "Children who need to be taught to respect traditional moral values are being taught that they have an inalienable right to be gay."[15] A year later she returned to the same theme: "Children need to be taught traditional moral values and to understand our religious heritage. We cannot leave them to discover for themselves what is right and wrong."[16] Indeed, the Prime Minister was "the driving force" behind Section 28, according to senior Government sources.[17]

Section 28 only makes sense according to a picture of human social and sexual relations in which everyone is basically heterosexual, save for a few inexplicable perverts, whose aim is to corrupt young people and seduce them into what is fondly described as "the gay lifestyle". One of the most decisive ways in which public AIDS commentary has changed the ideological field of British society is to be found in the widespread use of the notion of "the heterosexual community", in response to descriptions of how different communites of gay men and lesbians have responded to the epidemic. This new ideological unity is evidently primarily *defensive*. Hence the endless appeals to "tradition" and "heritage", which serve to replace those social institutions that have been widely sacrificed in the name of "self-sufficiency" and cost-cutting. Besides, Mrs Thatcher explicitly rejects the very idea of "the social". As far as she is concerned : "we've been through a period where too many people have been given to understand that if they have a problem, it's the government's job to cope with it. 'I have a problem, I'll get a grant.' 'I'm homeless, the government must house me.' They're casting their problem on society. And, you know, there is no such thing as society. There are individual men and women, and there are families. And no government can do anything except through people, and people must look to themselves first . . . A nation of free people will only continue to be great if family life continues and the structure of that nation is a family one."[18]

It is this dream-like fantasy of a nation which only exists as individuals in closed family units, supervised by government, that Thatcherism both draws on and wishes to impose with the full force of law. In this respect AIDS has played a central role in the ideological assault on all social values rooted in collectivities which are incompatible with this type of individualist absolutism. Michel Foucault and others have argued persuasively that modern forms of government authority depend increasingly on structures of political consent which involve strong personal identifications with institutions that are not necessarily recognized as "political". Thus governments may assume power in the name of "the family" or "the nation" or "traditional values", even and especially when these are presented as highly vulnerable and in need of "strong" action in order to protect them. Such abstract, ideological entities are presented as if they were natural phenomena, prior to and independent of the workings of state power. It is Foucault's contention that such categories, and the personal identities by which they are fleshed out and inhabited, are in fact indispensible mechanisms of state power itself, which he describes as the practice of "governmentality".[19] Of course, few people ever stop to consider why it is that they consent to state power and authority, except in moments of crisis. AIDS has been used to represent just such a crisis, pulling individuals round to identify *with* the government, in the name of "public health" and its protection. At the same time those who have actually been directly affected by AIDS are excluded from consideration as part of "the public" or "public health". Hence gay men in particular have suddenly found themselves not only politically unrepresented, but unable to discover any public institutions willing to acknowledge their only too real lived experience, including the routine denial of what are usually taken as fundamental social rights in the West — access to life insurance, mortgages, adequate social security, employment rights, and in many cases basic health care provision. After all, what is the place of gay men in relation to a National Health Service which has since its inception represented "the nation" and its health in exclusively heterosexual terms? How at this of all times are we to trust doctors who can write to their own professional journals asking if: "it is too much to hope for that homosexuality should be outlawed and that at least some sensible precautions should be taken to prevent the spread of AIDS to millions, even if those now relatively few victims of the disease need to suffer some deprivations to this end."[20] Or stating in a still more telling, and chilling metaphor, that: "I view homosexuals with the kind of vague loathing that I view terrorists."[21]

Eight years into the epidemic, the British government has still not spent a single penny on directly communicating support, sympathy or information to the social constituency that makes up more than 80 per cent of people with AIDS in the United Kingdom. We will only begin to understand this all but incredible state of affairs in relation to the specific forms of governmentality in modern Britain, and the obsessive mobilization of the *ideological* entities of family and nation. It goes without saying that most people with HIV infection and disease are officially regarded as if they are not members of families at all, a denial of reality fully backed up in law by the language of Section 28. This is largely a consequence of the historical institution of parliamentary democracy, which is by its nature deeply insensitive to the complex demographic make-up of the actual population of the UK. Parliament claims to stand for a pre-given "national interest" which assumes the existence of a unified homogeneous country, whilst at the same time: "it pre-empts all basic arguments about what the nation and its interests are and should be," as Raymond Williams has pointed out.[22]

For well over a century, parliamentarianism has successfully stifled the emergence of the types of popular politics rooted in notions of constitutional rights, which are so deeply constitutive of the political institutions and cultural identities of other European nations. British politics have rarely attempted to acknowledge the difficulties of addressing different population groups in Britain from a pluralist perspective. This is reflected in the strong resistance to constitutional reform, and the ways in which our archaic and profoundly undemocratic voting system, together with the bizarre assemblage of the House of Commons, the non-elected House of Lords, and the monarchy, are widely regarded as evidence of some imagined national superiority, rather than as sadly accurate indicators of our national political backwardness and chauvinism.

As Raymond Williams has pointed out, one result of parlia-mentarianism is that in political terms, "the whole range of social relations is reduced to two entities: the 'individual' and the 'nation'."[23] It is this principle that Mrs Thatcher has ruthlessly exploited, adding "the family" as the single central mediating term through which we are invited to make sense of ourselves and the world which, for better or worse, we are all obliged to share. It is precisely this dimension of sharing that is so glaringly absent from the Prime Minister's picture of life in contemporary Britain, where each family unit is supposedly entirely self-sufficient and cut off even from the next door neighbours. What is so striking about this vision of the ideal family unit is its sheer *loneliness* — the sense of imposed isolation, of frightened people peeping out nervously from behind the net curtains of respectability and supposedly universal "family values". It is against this desolate picture that we should pose David Edgar's sharp insight concerning the ways in which AIDS: "has brought into stark relief what many in the gay constituency knew already (particularly those who lived in gay communities), that a kinship based on shared nature and a consequent shared oppression can be as mutually sustaining as that of the family, and in many ways more binding and less conditional."[24]

Constructed on public hoardings and in newspaper and television adverts as an ideological "disease", the real complex tragedy of AIDS has been grotesquely exploited in order to bolster an ideologically powerful, cruelly narrow and punitive fantasy of family life. Yet we all know that marriages can go horribly and unexpectedly wrong. We know that parents and their children are not automatically compatible; that raising children is not a simple task to which everyone is "naturally" suited, and further, that not all family members are heterosexual. We also know that we do not consciously *choose* to be unhappy in our personal relationships, any more than we *choose* to get sick. These are the circumstances in which a yawning gulf may be recognized between the values and imperatives of "official" AIDS education, and campaigns organized by the communities that have actually been living with the reality of HIV infection and disease throughout the 1980s.

As narrow western theological proscriptions against homosexuality have gradually lost their authority, prejudice and cultural barriers remain strong, especially in countries like Britain where homosexuality has traditionally been exceptionally harshly treated by European standards. What is new to the twentieth century is the affirmation of a basic human right to consensual sexual expression, in the context of a wider intellectual and moral understanding of human sexuality as a field of rich diversity. Above all, it has been the emergence of the lesbian and gay movements, associated with Gay Liberation, which has transformed the lived experience of hundreds of thousands of British women and men, who have collectively rejected the insulting pathologized identity of "the homosexual", and come out as gay. The emergence of this gay movement in the United States, and Britain, and around the world, is one of the radical achievements of modern cultural politics. It is precisely this field of gay culture that is the principal target of so much contemporary concern. This is hardly surprising, since the values of gay culture are so profoundly incompatible with the narrow, pokey vision of the world, so eloquently defended by the Prime Minister. It is homosexuality which is increasingly being used to justify an entirely new set of political and ideological alignments, which pose the State as the supreme guarantor of "family values", now threatened not only by the "queers", but by what is presented as their viral surrogate, AIDS. It is therefore of crucial importance that we understand the language and values of official AIDS education materials in the light of the language and values of Section 28, which is not merely the most extreme example of explicitly anti-gay legislation seen anywhere in Europe since the notorious revision of paragraph 175 of the German penal code in 1935, which stated that *any* sexual act was punishable as a crime "if the inborn healthy instincts of the German people demand it."[25] It also arrives on top of the British AIDS epidemic, as a calculated insult to the lives of the thousand so far dead, and the thousands infected. Friends and colleagues who do not understand why we shake with rage when we hear the Prime Minister talk repeatedly about the "healthy instincts" of the British people evidently have a less developed acquaintance with recent European history.[26]

Disciplinary Versus Community-Based AIDS Education

Since the mid 1980s, local authorities throughout Britain have employed full-time HIV/AIDS educators to undertake local staff training, to liaise between different branches and sections of local government, to facilitate HIV/AIDS education in schools, health centres and the workplace, and to organize support services for those directly affected in the local community. Many of these new AIDS professionals have not come from the traditional backgrounds of health education and the social services, but gained their initial experience in the voluntary sector, working as volunteers with organizations such as the London Lesbian and Gay Switchboard, the Terrence Higgins Trust, Body Positive, and so on, which had faced the reality of AIDS long before the British government became involved. Since 1987 the government-sponsored National AIDS Trust has been delegated the responsibility of co-ordinating AIDS-related initiatives in the voluntary sector, and the Health Education Authority charged with the organization of AIDS education for the "general population". The huge voluntary sector response is entirely in keeping with the fashionable contemporary vision of self-help and non-dependance on state services. None the less, it is clear that the vast range of issues raised by the epidemic require central planning of some kind. The responsibility of government for public health and health care provision is still widely taken for granted in Britain.

Yet the communities affected first, and most severely, by the epidemic are evidently not officially regarded as members of the "public" in the same way that, for example, the citizens of Gloucestershire who recently faced a local meningitis outbreak were automatically understood to be a group with special and legitimate needs. Indeed, since very early in the history of the British HIV epidemic, "official" concern has been almost exclusively directed to the question of whether it would "spread" into what is usually described as the "general population" or, increasingly, as "the heterosexual community". This may be described as the ideology of "leakage", a favourite and significant term in such commentary. We have thus arrived at a situation where two almost entirely different approaches to "public" AIDS education co-exist:

one regarding "the public" as uninfected and exclusively heterosexual, the other conceiving the population as a complex matrix of
overlapping and interlocking social constituencies, all of which
contain infected members.

From early on in the history of the epidemic, non-government
AIDS service organizations struggled with little funding to produce
health education materials for gay men and injecting drug users, but
also for women as a whole, and for heterosexual men and young
people. Such organizations formed the first telephone advice lines,
and also provided local support services for those with HIV infection,
their friends, lovers and families. All this work has been entirely
dependent upon hundreds of thousands of hours of unpaid and
often thankless voluntary work each year, supported by charitable
fund-raising — almost exclusively from gay men at first — and small
one-off annual government grants, which make it impossible ever to
plan beyond a given twelve-month period. For example, the
Terrence Higgins Trust received £300,000 for the financial year
1988/89 from the Department of Health, paid belatedly with the
promise of an increase of a further £100,000 the following year. This
is less than one seventh of what the AIDS Action Committee of
Boston receives from American federal funds, for a city a quarter the
size of London. Furthermore the Trust is currently threatened with
an end to government funding in the early 1990s. Such a refusal to
learn from the catastrophic consequences of government under-
spending in the United States at a similar stage in the history of their
epidemic beggars belief. This is the immediate context in which we
must consider the different types of formal AIDS education in Britain.

Conventional biomedical health education distinguishes between
three types of preventative interventions: Primary Prevention, which
aims to minimize illness and disease amongst the well; Secondary
Prevention, which is concerned with the detection of disease, and
treatment care; and Tertiary Prevention, which is concerned with the
welfare of the chronically or terminally ill.[27] In these terms, national
government AIDS education strategy has been almost exclusively
involved with Primary Prevention, according to the ideological logic
of the Missionary Model of AIDS information, leaving the other two
areas to local government and non-government AIDS service
organizations. This is largely because government is unwilling or
unable to acknowledge those most immediately affected by HIV as

30   Simon Watney

members of an ideologically imagined "general public". It also
reveals an extraordinary and profoundly significant inability to
acknowledge and address the actual complexity and diversity of
sexual behaviour within what is posed as "the heterosexual
community". AIDS advertising sponsored by the Health Education
Authority demonstrates this with alarming clarity. For example, two
television advertisements shown on British television in 1988 both
aimed to show "casual sex" between previous strangers as "a bad
thing", something best avoided. In both ads, women are portrayed
as the "risk factor", luring "innocent" men to their doom. Both
implied that the men involved should not have sex with the women
they had met, and both therefore *ended* precisely where they should
have *begun*, with the question of how to have Safer Sex. For all
sexual relationships have to start somewhere, and who is to say what
constitutes "casual sex" and what constitutes the beginning of a
mutually satisfying relationship? It is in this context that we may
distinguish between AIDS education that is fundamentally congruent
with the Prime Minister's "vision" of a world drained of all
meaningful social and sexual relations beyond the family, and AIDS
education that addresses the actual circumstances in which most
women and men live and try to find happiness. These two
approaches are immediately evident when one compares AIDS
advertising produced by the government, and by the voluntary
sector.

A recent series of posters produced by the Terrence Higgins Trust
shows a series of pictures of gay men which are strongly erotic, and
aimed to reflect something of the diversity of gay culture and
sexuality. All share the same caption: "Safer Sex, Keep It Up!" with
the additional message, "antibody positive & negative — it's the
same for all." To begin with, it would be deeply insulting and
patronizing to produce Safer Sex materials for gay men which did
not respond to the fact that Safer Sex has been a commonplace for
several years. That does not mean that it is necessarily *easy*, and such
advertising aims to encourage and support many hundreds of
thousands of men in sustaining Safer Sex. In the real world it may be
relatively simple to have Safer Sex on a first encounter. But what
happens if a relationship follows, if two people fall in love? What
happens after six weeks, or six months, or six *years?* We need to
affirm the passion of sex and the force of desire. This is not
helped by the type of Safer Sex publicity that talks casually about

"non-penetrative sex", as if penetration were not a *fundamental* aspect of the psychic meaning of human sexuality. This is a particularly important question for gay men who like to fuck and to be fucked, and who have often had to overcome very powerful cultural taboos in order to accept their own sexuality. The Trust's advertising has a relatively limited aim — to keep the subject of Safer Sex "in the air", to recognize that HIV is an issue which affects an entire complex network of gay communities, and to affirm the irreducible value and importance of our common human sexuality. It also insists that Safer Sex is an issue for *all* gay men, regardless of antibody status. From this perspective, HIV is not regarded as something which is somebody else's problem and responsibility, but a reality which must be faced *collectively.* After all, most gay men who were sexually active in the late 1970s and early 1980s recognize that there is a high possibility that they may already be infected. HIV education amongst gay men therefore seeks to support people in an unprecedented situation, and to repeat the message that HIV is not just something one might "catch" from somebody else, but is something that one might be equally likely to give to another person. In this respect, such community-based advertising calls into question the whole set of distinctions between Primary, Secondary and Tertiary health education strategies, since it regards people with HIV infection and disease as a central part of the gay community, as real people with real social and sexual needs, just like everybody else.

This approach could hardly be more different from the newspaper-based campaign launched by the Health Education Authority (HEA) in December 1988, with the by-line: "AIDS. You're As Safe As You Want To Be." The "you" in this campaign is an isolated individual, whom, it seems, can only be *frightened* into Safer Sex. The first advert in the series of four asks in large white letters, against a stark black background: "What Is the Difference Between HIV and AIDS?", with the one-word reply, "Time". This is hardly the way to establish the distinction between a virus with clearly established modes of transmission, and a syndrome. Nor is it technically correct, since even the most pessimistic medical evidence only places the average progression at between 75 and 90 per cent.[28] In any case, it runs counter to all established health education principles to tell people they are simply going to die, without any kind of accompanying counselling, as one would hope to find in a proper patient-doctor relationship. HIV has effectively been telescoped into AIDS, with the "information" that: "Obviously, the more people you sleep with the more likely you are to become infected. But the answer doesn't just mean fewer sexual partners. It also means using a condom, or even having sex that avoids penetration. AIDS may be incurable but it's also avoidable."

This is in fact an extraordinary confection of euphemism and plain misinformation. The number of one's sexual partners can only be counted as a risk factor for HIV if one is having unsafe sex. The adverts thus immediately offer a conflicting message between the issue of *numbers* of sexual partners, and of the *type* of sex one has. This is particularly dangerous since it implies that HIV is not a potential risk, for example, to someone who has only had sex with one or two people in the last decade. It also implies that there is an *alternative* to Safer Sex. However, as one American doctor wrote recently: "AIDS is here to stay. It is like the day after Hiroshima — the world has changed and will never be the same again."[29] She also points out with admirable directness that: "There has never been a society in which the patterns of sexual behaviour were restricted solely to monogamy or chastity, and America [or Britain] . . . is not going to be the first."[30]

Another advert in the HEA series takes up two pages, the first simply showing a small photograph of a head and shoulders, its features obliterated by heavy shadow, in the traditional convention of the anonymous criminal, with the caption: "For This Many People With AIDS" — answered on the next page by — "This Many People Have The Virus", set beneath six rows of five similarly blacked out faces. The overall campaign is evidently trying to make up for the previous four years in which no "public" health education materials had ever taken the trouble to distinguish between HIV and AIDS, save by totally misleading references to the so-called "AIDS virus". It is not however clear that the latest campaign really improves on its predecessors, since the small print which contains all the information is totally dominated by the images and headline questions. This is most troubling in another advert which asks: "If AIDS Only Affects 0.002% Of The Population Why Is This Advertisement Appearing In Every National Newspaper?". Why indeed, one, might ask, since readers who cannot acknowledge that they may be at risk are unlikely to consult the microscopic "explanation" underneath the question. At the same time, the dramatic emphasis on AIDS statistics, without HIV figures, can only serve to *obscure* the importance and significance of attempts to distinguish between the two.

Throughout the entire campaign, people with HIV infection or disease appear only as anonymous deterrents, rather than people who need to be seen as very much like any newspaper readers — as ordinary people. This is clearly because at some basic level they are not regarded in such a way by the advertising agency, or the HEA. Such advertisements take us on an extraordinary Gulliver's Travels through the unconscious sexual anxieties aroused by the epidemic, calling up a galaxy of strange and frightening types of people, from "prostitutes" and "the promiscuous" to "drug abusers" and "bi-sexuals". Such campaigns clearly demonstrate that: "Throughout the ages, we can see not a one-way dependency but interplay and exchange between scientific and non-scientific modes of thought."[31] It is evident that the ideological Terrorist and Missionary inter-pretations of AIDS which permeate popular culture are equally felt as powerful forces on both medical attitudes and health education involved with HIV, and in all areas of "professional" commentary on the epidemic.

This is perhaps most apparent in the routine reporting practices of professional journalists, who are positioned between their readers and sources of information, which range from medical journals, international conferences, and press releases from government bodies such as the Department of Health and the HEA. There has been almost no serious investigative journalism into the political dimensions of the British HIV epidemic outside the gay press, which might as well be published on another planet as far as the national weeklies and dailies are concerned.[32] "Human interest" criteria may make space for pathos-laden stories concerning "AIDS victims", as long as they happen to be heterosexual. Hence the regular "Tragic AIDS Family" stories, which recast the Terrorist and Missionary models' interpretation of the epidemic into individual narratives, with which readers are invited to identify. I have not read a single feature in the British press which treats a gay man with HIV as part of a biological or an extended family. Nor have I come across a single feature concerning the availability of treatment drugs, the ethics of placebo trials, or the wider medical politics of organizations working on behalf of people with HIV infection or disease. The image of HIV as a uniformly fatal condition requires an emphasis on biomedical issues that restricts concern either to questions of alleged culpability on the part of infected individuals ("AIDS carriers"), or the fantasy of a "cure" or vaccine. Without a clear distinction between HIV and AIDS, there can be no consideration of early interventions, or recognition that there can never be a single all-purpose cure for the syndrome, given the wide range of conditions that collectively constitute AIDS. Nor can there be any acknowledgement that many of these conditions are individually preventable or curable. Given that most journalists writing about the epidemic have been doing so for several years, this is a sorry reflection of the values and news criteria of the British press.

To take just one example: Clare Dover has been writing about AIDS in the *Daily Express* for some time as its medical reporter. Her work is certainly not the best, nor by any stretch of the imagination the worst in the field of "AIDS journalism". It is the very typicality of her work that makes it significant. In December 1988 she described a World AIDS Day conference which had taken place in London, as part of an international event sponsored by the World Heath Organization. Needless to say, the international dimension went entirely unremarked. Her article ran under the headline: "Britain's £1bn AIDS Bill", with a supplementary rider stating that: "Health Minister Mellor Pledges Big Cash Boost in Battle To Beat The Disease."[33] There was also a smaller column heading: "Hope For Babies", and a list of numbered statements under a heading printed white on black: "20 Facts You Need To Know About A Killer." It may prove useful to run through this story in some detail, since it epitomizes British press coverage of the epidemic.

Initially, the article focuses on the possible financial costs of the epidemic: "Britain could face a bill or more than £1 billion to treat the hundreds of thousands of people infected by AIDS in 1992." The official government estimate of "30,000 cases by 1992" is then contrasted with the figure of "100,000 to 300,000 who could be infected", according to Professor Michael Adler, from London's Middlesex Hospital. There is an immediate confusion between HIV statistics and those of AIDS, with the former presented as the latter. The key word in this slippage is "cases": thus people with HIV simply become "AIDS victims". Nor is the astonishing disparity between the two sets of figures commented upon. Instead, Dover rushes forward to describe how the Minister of Health has : "pledged a further £14 million next year to help health authorities develop local initiatives to prevent the spread. Target groups will include homosexual and bisexual men, drug misusers, prostitutes and their clients, and people attending clinics for sexually transmitted diseases."

Through all of this, the primary focus is evidently financial, and the story makes no sense at all unless we are able to decipher its sub-text, which tells us that "we", the readers of the *Daily Express*, are going to have to shell out vast sums of "our" money to pay for the medical consequences of "other people's" sexual permissiveness and perversion. Risk and responsibility are firmly located with the named "target groups", whose own responses to the epidemic are never considered. Since they are not regarded as constituent parts of the nation, it follows that they must be closely policed by "health authorities" in the form of "local initiatives", whatever that might entail. Nor is there any acknowledgement that these same "target groups" have been in the foreground of HIV/AIDS education since the beginning of the epidemic, and were working on behalf of the rest of the population long before the government or any of its agencies become involved. On the contrary, significant sections of the British press are clearly hostile to HIV/AIDS education developed by and for such groups. Hence the lengthy attack in the *Sunday Telegraph* on the work of the Terrence Higgins Trust on the grounds that it is "a homosexual conspiracy", a view which is regularly repeated in *The Sunday Times* and *The Observer*, where Richard Ingrams writes the most homophobic column in Britain.[34] HIV education must at any cost be made to conform with the dominant moral agenda shared by the government and the press. Hence the decision by Leicester police to prevent the distribution of a Safer Sex leaflet for local prostitutes, drawn up by the women themselves, with funding from the city council.[35]

Furthermore, there is no sense whatsoever of the implications of the statistics being tossed around as casually as if they referred to the annual export figures for helicopters. Yet these same figures reveal that perhaps three hundred thousand people in Britain will have contracted HIV by 1992. Nothing could tell us more about the contemporary "politics of the family" than this *total* disregard for the sheer enormity of the human tragedy of HIV. It is as if the story of the Pan-Am jumbo jet which crashed onto the small Scottish town of Lockerbie in December 1988, with the loss of less than one hundredth of these figures in human lives, had been written up in terms of the "scandalous" cost to the local fire-brigade and mortuary attendants of clearing up the remains of "alien" Americans who had only themselves to blame for having had the temerity to fly at an altitude of six miles in the first place, knowing the risks . . . Those who lost their lives on the ground would of course be treated as "innocent victims", unless they were discovered to have had HIV, in which circumstance they would become "deadly AIDS carriers", putting "our boys" at risk, as one man who lost his life trying to save others in the King's Cross underground station fire was described by the *Daily Mail.*[36] Nothing persuades me that the basic elements of the ideological agenda determining the coverage of AIDS in the British media have significantly changed in the course of the past five years, or that the "target groups" listed here are not still widely regarded as disposable in their entirety.[37] Suggestions that an early "over-reaction" has been followed by a subsequent "under-reaction" entirely miss the point of an underlying consistency of attitudes which inform the major Britain institutions that "handle" and frame public opinion.

The solitary note of optimisim in the story concerned the "Hope For Babies", with a report that three out of four infants born to "AIDS-infected mothers" will "never develop the disease themselves". This is entirely in contrast with the "20 Facts You Need To Know About A Killer", which immediately places the entire subject of HIV within a homicidal frame of reference, according to which people with HIV infection or disease, rather than the virus itself, are seen as killers. The list provides what amounts to a detailed miniature circuit-diagram of the unconscious workings of AIDS ideology, with most of its systematic confusions, contradictions, omissions, elisions, and denials. It may therefore prove helpful to go through the twenty points, in order to clarify the ways in which such commentary constitutes a "general knowledge" of AIDS which by mis-informing has the potential to do much harm.

1. "The virus is thought to have arisen in Africa, but now millions of people are infected worldwide." The initial issue here is the relation between the *source* of HIV, and its supposed *cause.*[38] This is the decisive ideological mechanism by which disease is interpreted as punishment, with symptoms regarded as signs which reveal some secret guilt on the part of the diseased, who can thus be conveniently identified as the "guilty ones", to be blamed for their own condition, and still more so for that of their "innocent" victims.

A heavily fantasized "central Africa" is conjured up in such commentary as the location of this primal responsibility. Epidemiologists do not agree that HIV necessarily originated anywhere on the continent of Africa, but in any case the Africa of such assertions is not so much a geographical as an ideological location, hence its distinctive vagueness, making the epidemic "knowable" in terms of a long racist legacy of colonial connotations of supposed depravity, dirt and disease. These permit a two-way ideological traffic between an unhygienic Africa, imagined as the original cesspool of disease, and an equally unhygienic homosexuality, similarly understood as a "natural" source of contagion — both medically and sexually "unhealthy." In this manner "African AIDS" becomes another version of "the white man's burden", rather than a catastrophe for Africans themselves, who are reduced to the status of potential "AIDS carriers".[39]

2. "It was brought to Haiti, where gay Americans descended in droves for cheap sex with cash-hungry rent boys." The "it" here is HIV, though how and when "it" was supposedly brought to Haiti is far from clear. Suffice to say that from the perspective of the Terrorist model, the epidemic is pictured as a kind of relay race, with the virus as a deadly baton being handed on from one "target group" to another. AIDS ideology contains a limited cast of character types, which emerged very early in Western reporting of the epidemic, and have proved highly resistant to modification of any kind. Thus "prostitutes", "Haitians", "gay men", "Africans", "drug addicts" and so on have to be related to one another via narrative fantasies which tell us much about the unconscious of professional journalism, and nothing about actual epidemiology. Thus Haitian society is reconstructed in the likeness of the tabloids' view of Britain, complete with "rent boys", a specifically British term for male prostitutes. Yet when transposed to the exotic "voodoo" world of Haiti, they magically become the (almost) innocent "victims" of the "gay Americans" who "descended" in vulture-like "droves". Yet it is these same Americans who are supposedly getting infected by the Haitian "rent boys", whose depiction as "cash-hungry" subtly confuses motives of poverty with those of greed. There is of course no question of there being such a person as a young gay Haitian. In this manner the "gay Americans" and the "rent boys" are presented as mutually victimizing, in such a way that there is no danger of our

making any kind of sympathetic identification with either group.[40] The Americans are made to seem to get their just deserts as paedophile sex tourists, out for "cheap sex", whilst the "rent boys" become greedy, murderous "AIDS carriers". Yet it is always painfully apparent to gay readers that this type of "exposure" journalism disavows just the kind of "holiday fun" that is gleefully celebrated in the same publications every summer — as long as it's "healthily" heterosexual, and taking place on the Costa Del Sol. AIDS must therefore be rigorously homosexualized and distanced, in order not to threaten such unimpeachable pleasures. Such confusions and contradictions are deeply telling of British press attitudes towards sexuality in general, and homosexuality in particular, and nowhere more so than in relation to the highly ambiguous figure of the "rent boy", who combines the cultural attributes of both the voracious seasoned prostitute and "innocent" youth. It is frequently difficult to decide which is considered the more seductive characteristic. Rent boys are habitually constructed in this revealingly ambivalent fashion, embodying the ever potent fantasy of the sexually predatory adolescent, who must be punished for awakening the repressed desire of "vulnerable" adults. The precise degree of punishment meted out to them by journalists is an exact index of levels of social and psychological resistance to male sexual memories, of which the "rent boy" is a displaced substitute. Thus, whether British or Haitian, the "rent boy" may be anything from fifteen to forty, as long as he has a good juicy scandal to sell concerning some older celebrity, or better still, gay men as a whole. In this context, we should not overlook the significance of regarding "gay men" as a fixed, *quantifiable* minority, which conveniently overlooks the fluidity of sexual behaviour and identities for individuals and the whole population.[41]

3. "They took it back to San Francisco and New York, where homosexual promiscuity was being flaunted." Here the Missionary model is in control, according to which homosexuality is intrinsically "promiscuous" since unsanctioned by marriage. The same centrifugal force of familial ideology that flings gay men and lesbians out from the confines of "the family" and "the nation" must also be on constant guard against their continued external threat to "real" families. Thus any affirmation of homosexuality as other than a shameful personal secret, is interpreted as "flaunting", in just the

same way that Section 28 interprets any positive representation of lesbians or gay men as "promoting" homosexuality. "Promiscuity" is the pivotal word here, calling on the official message that HIV is somehow a direct result of the numbers of one's sexual partners, regardless of sexual practices. Familialism reveals its terror of consensual sexual pleasure most clearly in its obsessive rhetorical concern with numbers of sexual partners, at the expense of Safer Sex information. People must at all costs be protected from the frightening possibility of choice in sexual matters, which is presented as literally fatal.

4. "The homosexuals lit the powderkeg and the first blast rebounded on themselves." Here the homosexualization of HIV is metaphorically linked with connotations of terrorism in the familiar rhetoric of reporting actual events, when bombers accidentally blow themselves up. The Princess Royal was speaking from this same position when she described AIDS as: "a classic own goal, scored by the human race on itself," when she opened the World Health Organization's Global AIDS Summit in London in January 1988. The rush of British journalists to defend her words shows their significance.[42] At the same time, the imagery keys in with the widespread notion of people with HIV as "living time-bombs" which has prevailed for many years, and is internalized by many gay men themselves.[43]

5. "Anal sex is not how nature designed the human anatomy, and resulting injuries enable the virus to get quickly into the blood-stream." At this point an overwhelming biologistic functionalism is brought into play, as the "20 Facts" move on from gay men to heterosexuals. The unconscious message seems to be that unprotected anal sex is the main risk factor for HIV transmission, and by avoiding it, readers will be safe. Needless to say, there is no suggestion of using a condom for anal sex, since an exact correspondence is being established between "acts" and "disease". This is reinforced in the alarming language of "injuries", invoked as a graphic warning against forbidden pleasures.[44]

6. "Everyone, apart from those who are faithful to long-term partners, is in danger." This presumably means that even long-term gay relationships are safe, though this is hardly what is intended. Nor

does it take adequate account of the average time delay between HIV infection and diagnosable symptoms. How long is "long-term"? Once again, the Missionary model refuses to allow Safer Sex information which might take heed of the diversity of actual sexual practices. We are thus offered a metaphysical or magical solution to HIV infection in the form of marriage, or at least monogamy.

7. "Bisexuals take it home to their wives. Needle-sharing drug addicts pass it on with dirty needles. As addicts are heterosexual, their sex partners and those who sleep with them are at risk." Two fascinating assumptions coincide here: first, that all bisexuals are male, and second that all injecting drug users are heterosexual. We thus move directly from the implication that there is little risk of infection, to the implication that risk is potentially everywhere. Such starkly conflicting messages are entirely in keeping with the overall tendency of the British press to veer constantly from one extreme to the other in relation to the question of heterosexual transmission.[45]

8. "International studies indicate that men with the virus have a 15 to 20 per cent chance of infecting their wives." Again, questions of Safer Sex are absent from this picture of an abstract degree of risk, which, even if it were empirically demonstrated — which it is not — would not be predictive either for individuals or for married couples. The issue of female-to-male transmission is simply ignored, as perhaps too dreadful to contemplate.

9. "The risk of passing it on through 'straight' sex is considerably lower than through gay sex." Clare Dover had evidently changed her mind in the four weeks since she had reported that: "Thousands of people have already caught AIDS through normal sex," noting that: "In Africa, the disease hits men and women equally, and unprotected sex is the means of spread."[46] At the same time "sex" is understood as unprotected fucking, whatever the gender of the people involved. Yet again, Safer Sex is simply ignored, and "gay sex" presented as if it were an *intrinsic* risk factor, regardless of what gay men actually do sexually.

10. "The virus is more easily passed on when the sex partner has just picked up the infection, or is just about to become ill with AIDS." This certainly tallies with the most recent evidence, though it

is difficult to imagine what most readers would make of this information, since nothing has previously prepared them in the course of the article — or any of Clare Dover's earlier reports — for such a significant distinction between the virus and the syndrome.[47]

11. "Men with haemophilia who become infected with AIDS through their treatment tend not to pass on the infection to their wives." It would appear that the entire significance of the previous point has been ignored. The implication remains that risk is determined by the gender of sexual partners, rather than the natural history of HIV, which the most recent evidence strongly suggests is most infectious shortly after transmission and, again, late in the history of HIV disease.

12. "Despite all the falling tombstone advertisements, homo-sexuals only started to change their habits when they saw friends dying." This is gratuitously insulting, since it flies in the face of the worldwide evidence concerning the adoption of Safer Sex by gay men in the early stages of the epidemic.[48] Gay men cannot be seen to be setting an example. At this point we may detect a certain anxiety emerging, as if Safer Sex is somehow itself a form of homosexuality. Certainly right-wing critics of Safer Sex materials for gay men are in no doubt that these "promote" homosexuality.[49] Such attitudes bear out Cindy Patton's observation that heterosexuals are generally presented as having a *right* to know about HIV, whereas gay men have a *responsibility* to know. This is consistent with the general tenor of revenge fantasies concerning those deemed to be responsible for HIV. Hence the cruelty of so much AIDS commentary, which is entirely congruent with the punitive imperative to prevent any kind of sympathetic identification with those most immediately devastated by the epidemic.

13. "The rate of spread among homosexuals is falling." Any amplification on this laconic statement would require a mention of Safer Sex practices. Heterosexuals must evidently be protected from any information about how gay men have responded to the epidemic. Gay men must not be seen as caring communities, but only as individual perverts. Moverover, Safer Sex has the incon-venience of drawing attention to the fact that all forms of human sexuality are much of a muchness.

14. "The spread among drug addicts is increasing. Now 26 per cent of addicts tested at one West London clinic were infected." Without any information concerning when or where these "drug addicts" were infected, such figures remain meaningless. At the same time, responsibility for being infected is placed onto injecting drug users, rather than state policies which have made syringes increasingly difficult to get hold of, as a direct result of the de-medicalization and consequent re-criminalization of all aspects of injecting drug use. Nor is there any acknowledgement of the equally serious problem of the one-off injecting drug user, perhaps sharing a needle at a party for kicks, or for a dare, or whatever. References to "drug addicts" or "drug misusers" bear little relation to the actual complexity of drug use in the real world.

15. "One in 100 people who claim they are heterosexuals attending London sexually transmitted disease clinics is HIV positive." This is a particularly transparent example of the wish to disavow heterosexual transmission, since it carries the strong implication that many of these "heterosexuals" are in fact gay or bisexual. If as may indeed be the case, some bisexuals, gay men and lesbians feel the need to pass as heterosexuals this may reflect the increasing hostility of mass media reporting.[50]

16. "By the end of last year 20,000 to 50,000 people were infected. This includes 13,000 to 30,000 homosexual men and 2,000 to 5,500 sworn heterosexuals." In fact, official British epidemiological statistics listed a total of 1598 cases of AIDS in the UK up to 30 June 1988, and 8,794 people with HIV.[51] Such figures are undoubtedly on the low side, given the strong legal and cultural disincentives to voluntary HIV testing which prevail in Britain, but they do at least serve to reveal the fanciful nature of Ms Dover's claims. The category of the "sworn heterosexual" is however of some significance, since it is most unlikely that anyone would disbelieve the sexual identity of a self-describing gay man.

17. "As most injecting drug misusers and haemophiliacs are heterosexual, 6,000 to 17,000 heterosexuals could be infected." Somewhere between here and point 7, the unqualified statement that "addicts are heterosexual" has evidently been forgotten. As for the figures, they are as reliable as any other speculations.[52]

18. "It takes an average of eight years between picking up the virus and becoming ill." This average conforms with the most recent figures from the US Centers for Disease Control, but once more, it needs to be pointed out that such statistics are never *predictive* for individuals. We should also note the way in which the distinction between HIV infection and disease is ignored, emphasized, forgotten, and then picked up again.

19. "HIV is the deadliest virus the world has ever seen, killing 80 per cent or more of those it infects." The consensus of biomedical opinion currently places the rate of progression from HIV infection to disease at between 75 and 90 per cent.[53] It should however be pointed out that there is no empirical evidence to confirm that HIV disease ("AIDS") is invariably fatal, and as I have repeatedly stressed, most individual symptoms are either preventable or treatable.

20. "There is no vaccine and no cure." Here we find the ne plus ultra of AIDS "education", totally uninterested in the wide varieties of clinical treatment interventions, and other non-medical therapies. The word AIDS itself is not even needed, as for those Americans who prefer to talk euphemistically of "the A word" rather than acknowledge a painful and constantly changing reality.

The immense convenience of this epidemic in providing a seeming "justification" for cranks, and moralistic bigots, to tout their vulgar nostrums with total impunity cannot be over-emphasized. Ignoring all medical evidence, and flouting the most basic notions of consideration and responsibility, such journalism provides an encouragement for still more blatant misinterpretation. Hence, for example, the words of influential right-wing politician Sir Alfred Sherman in a letter to *The Times*, challenging a liberal "AIDS charter" financed by the HEA attacking the stigmatization of people with HIV, and signed by numerous celebrities. Sherman was "affronted", since people with AIDS are: "mainly sodomites and drug-abusers, together with numbers of women who voluntarily associate with this sexual underworld."[54] Such attitudes tend to place the speaker above any possible personal risk. Moreover it is clear that heterosexual men are somehow regarded as the only "innocent" category, though surrounded on all sides by the dreadful creatures of the "sexual underworld". By localizing AIDS as primarily within this "underworld", Sherman and others draw attention away from the importance of Safer Sex for everyone. Resistance to Safer Sex is not the prerogative of men, as British research has shown.[55] Sherman concludes that : "We seek their redemption for which remorse and repentance are a sine qua non."[56] Such claims to a moral high-ground from which to judge others plainly articulates the primarily disciplinary motives which inform most "official" government attitudes to HIV. These connect a profound dread of and contempt for the sick, with a deep-seated fear and loathing of all that escapes the comprehension of those for whom there is no social world beyond the individual and "the family". Not far beneath the conscious, explicit level of belief that informs the HEA campaign, Sir Alfred Sherman's letter, and countless thousands of articles and TV programmes like it, there lies a hatred so fierce and so cruel that it is casually prepared to deny any kind of genuinely helpful information about HIV to those regarded as "enemies" of the national family unit. The underlying punitive and sadistic fantasy of AIDS as a uniformly disfiguring, agonizing, and untreatable fatal condition, expresses a gloating wish-fulfilment fantasy which I can acknowledge, but which is too painful for me to dwell upon in the detail it deserves.

From Ideology to Practice, From Practice to Resistance

Beyond the field of clinical diagnosis, AIDS is primarily an ideological term which condenses all aspects of HIV infection and disease into a single entity. As such, AIDS draws upon and unifies a wide range of social attitudes, beliefs and fears. This is nowhere more obvious than in the continuing dispute over the concept of the "AIDS victim", a term which was first coherently and collectively refused at the second US AIDS forum, held in Denver, Colorado, in 1983. This founding statement of people with AIDS/ARC, widely known as "The Denver Principles", states simply: "We condemn attempts to label us as 'victims', which implies defeat, and we are only occasionally 'patients', which implies passivity, helplessness and dependence upon the care of others. We are 'people with AIDS'."[57] In spite of much discussion in the press, the term "AIDS victim" is still the most frequently used term in Britain and the US, sometimes modified to "AIDS sufferer". Both terms are used to describe people with HIV as well as people with AIDS, a confusion which is repeated and reinforced in the equally common use of the term "AIDS-carrier".[58] The use of such terms as "drug addict" and "drug abuser" implies a distance from the experience of HIV infected drug users, and from an understanding of community-based AIDS education.

Yet the ways in which we talk about HIV infection and disease are not necessarily always the same, but may change with context. For example, it is frequently helpful in elementary AIDS education to relate the situation of people with HIV to that of others living with chronic disease in the community. Given the relatively brief periods of time that most people with HIV disease spend in hospital, it should be stressed that HIV is very much an issue for community medicine and community services, including social workers, psychiatric social workers, meals on wheels, continence advisers, and so on. It is also important to emphasize the ways in which such community-care services have suffered in recent years, together with emergency housing facilities, and other emergency welfare services, on which most chronically sick people depend so heavily. At other times however, it can be equally important to establish those aspects of HIV which are sui generis, from the types of stress to which people with HIV are sadly often subjected as a direct effect of AIDS ideology, to specific biomedical issues, including the question of treatment and the availability of therapeutic drugs.

HIV is increasingly regarded by doctors and other health and care providers as a manageable condition, and the average life expectancy of people with HIV disease has risen dramatically with the gradually increased availability of drug treatments, especially in the United States, where far more drug trials are underway than in Britain, although they are often only available to those who are sufficiently well insured, or who can afford them privately. No aspect of the HIV epidemic is more fraught with controversy than the subject of drug trials. A thoroughly bad precedent was set as long ago as September 1986, when Burroughs-Wellcome "launched" AZT at an American press conference without even bothering to establish any protocols concerning how doctors or people with HIV might get hold of it, or the criteria for eligibility. Such grotesque insensitivity is still unfortunately characteristic of most reporting of new drugs. To begin with, we must distinguish between different kinds of available drugs. First, there are antivirals, which are intended to retard HIV disease by preventing the replication of the virus. Secondly, there are immune stimulants, which are intended to support or rebuild the damaged immune system. Thirdly, there are prophylactic drugs, intended to prevent the occurrence or recurrence of individual HIV related conditions, such as PCP. It is extremely bewildering for doctors and people with HIV alike that there is still no reliable international list of ongoing drug trials, with information concerning how many people are enrolled, dates of commencement, and so on. There should as an absolute priority be a national AIDS data bank, open to everyone, which would show, for example, which drugs look most promising, which trials exclude women, which are taking place in the developing world, and so on. Unfortunately the high potential profitability of such drugs encourages secrecy and the raising of prices by the private pharmaceutical industry, on which both private and socialized medicine are equally dependent. This means in effect that many HIV related drugs are least available to those most in need.

In the absence of a national AIDS data bank with full access to the latest international information, many people with HIV in Britain are following the example of the United States, where "guerrilla clinics" and "buyers' clubs" have flourished for several years, providing people with drugs known to have no harmful consequences, yet unavailable to them. There is a serious ethical problem here. As Dr Mathilde Krim, founding chair of the American Foundation for AIDS Research (AmFAR) has argued: "Drug development has been very slow. We have tens of thousands of people sick with terminal disease in this country, and only 2,900 of them in government clinical trials. That's not very many..."[59] The use of placebos in such trials is equally worrying, and can only be explained in relation to an AIDS ideology which justifies breaches of conventional medical ethics by analogy with the "special case" of a war-time situation.[60] Thus for example a Medical Research Council sponsored trial of AZT as a possibly effective early intervention drug for people with HIV infection who have not developed serious disease is currently underway in Britain, with a thousand clients, scattered around thirty different medical centres. Of these, five hundred will only receive a placebo.

In such circumstances we must insist that all drug trials be regarded as forms of medical treatment too. Our first priority should be the proper management of people with HIV, who do not simply develop disease out of the blue. Many people with HIV develop medical conditions that are either preventable or treatable, if they are receiving regular evaluations in the form of blood tests which can detect the characteristic and well-known abnormalities that predict the onset of HIV disease. We need only consider the situation of a newly diagnosed person with HIV whose blood tests indicate that she has a 59 per cent chance of developing HIV related disease within two years, and who is at the same time only offered the opportunity to enter the MRC trial of AZT, on which she has a fifty-fifty chance of only getting a sugar-pill placebo for the next three years. Yet this is the only treatment drug trial being financed by the MRC, from a 1988–1992 research budget of £26.5 million! In this respect, the priorities of "official" biochemical research directly reflect the imperatives of AIDS ideology. Scientific attention is almost exclusivly directed to the search for a vaccine against HIV infection, and is fatalistic in regard to the situation of those who are actually infected. The failure to fund research into treatment initiatives for people with HIV is perhaps the clearest indicator of the workings of AIDS ideology in the field of professional biomedicine, and of the stark division between the priorities of "pure science" researchers working far away from the epidemic, and those of physicians working directly in the front line of patient management and care.

In the United Kingdom we lack the types of national civil rights organizations that exist in the United States, which act both as powerful advocates and as models for the emergence of new, specifically AIDS related organizations. Of these, by far the most important has been the AIDS Coalition To Unleash Power (ACT UP), which has generated an unprecedented activist politics, dedicated to exposing the appalling circumstances of most people with HIV infection and disease in the USA.[61] Here in Britain we must expect the emergence of a similar direct response to both the ideology of AIDS, and the practices that it encourages and validates. This will involve strategic interventions at the levels of public representation and commentary, in order to challenge and undermine the "official" ideology of AIDS, and to re-present the entire meaning and significance of the epidemic. It will also require strategic inter-ventions in relation to the institutions that are directly responsible for managing the epidemic — from the Department of Health, and the Health Education Authority, to teaching hospitals, the media, the British Medical Association, the insurance industry, and so on. This project is the cultural politics of AIDS.

Conclusion: The Cultural Politics of AIDS
These days one can *hear* the HIV epidemic in cities such as New

York and San Francisco, in the form of the regular four-hourly bleepers that sound everywhere, in restaurants, cinemas and theatres, reminding people to take their drugs. The epidemic is also clearly visible, as the result of the wholesale fly-posting by ACT UP of entire cities with their Silence=Death Stickers, and their overnight responses to the latest AIDS scandal. In the context of the catastrophic consequences of private medicine, ACT UP has been primarily involved with the issue of experimental drugs and drug treatment provision, together with directly AIDS related discrimination. At the same time cities such as New York have developed a huge network of cultural responses, ranging from fund raising benefits to installations such as ACT UP's "Let the Record Show" in the Broadway window of the New Museum. The American cultural response has been admirably summarized by Douglas Crimp in his introduction to the special issue of *October* magazine on "AIDS : Cultural Analysis, Cultural Activism."[62]

Here in Britain we are faced with a rather different situation, where it is necessary to construct a cultural politics that is able to address the three closely related issues of political representation, cultural representations, and HIV related health care provision and services. This involves a co-ordinated critique of parliamentarianism as such, and its attendant institutions, including parliamentary press correspondents, party politics, and civil rights organizations such as Amnesty International, which has consistently refused to consider the political situation of lesbians and gay men. It also involves a co-ordinated critique of systems and institutions controlling "public" representations, as well as creating a specific culture of AIDS which could effectively take apart the dominant cultural agenda of "official" AIDS ideology, as expressed in the Terrorist and Missionary Models.[63] Lastly, it involves a co-ordinated critique of the institutions of medicine, welfare, health education, the rehabilitation of drug users, the police, and so on. This is an enormously ambitious project, which will require large numbers of people from many different backgrounds, with many different skills. It will be necessary to construct a symbolic politics that can provide a more adequate and convincing way for most people to understand the situation of people with HIV infection and disease, together with their communities, following the magnificent example of ACT UP in the assertion that: "We are a diverse non-partisan group of people committed to direct action to end the AIDS crisis."[64]

We cannot accept the dominant image of people with HIV as totally isolated, pathetic, silent, hospitalized, dying "AIDS victims". We have to transform the terms in which AIDS is *thought* (and feared, and dreaded, and made the stuff of countless nightmares, or entirely disavowed), in order to improve the circumstances in which people with HIV live. This means taking liberties in every sense of those words. It means taking to the streets, and taking control of our lives, and asserting liberties which no virus or government can ever completely deny us. This will require negotiations, and dialogue, and alliances between social groups that are in many respects profoundly disparate, including injecting drug users, people of colour, lesbians, and gay men, doctors and nurses, teachers, trades unionists, and many others. If HIV has brought out all that is most sordid and squalid in British culture and society, our response must bring out all that is best. The quality of mercy in modern Britain is threatened, with newspapers read daily by millions calling for "leper-like colonies" on the grounds that "the human race is under threat" from "promiscuous homosexuals" who "are by far the biggest spawning ground for AIDS."[65] We live under a government which the Prime Minister herself has described as a "regime", supported by one of the least democratic newspaper industries in the Western world. Nadezhda Mandelstam wrote that: "People living under a dictatorship are soon filled with a sense of their helplessness, in which they find an excuse for their own passivity."[66] Strangely her words have a grim resonance in contemporary Britain. Yet it is precisely that passivity that our cultural politics must be able to reach and awaken.

Such a project cannot afford to proceed from the assumption that the issues and dilemmas we face are intrinsically newsworthy. On the contrary, the public representation of most people affected by HIV is already subject to the most rigorous ideological policing, as we have seen. This is precisely why we have to understand the rules and conventions that establish "newsworthiness", and govern public visibility and audibility, in order to be able to manipulate the mass media in ways that will guarantee that we are seen and heard on TV and in the press on our terms, rather than those of an industry which invariably frames us either as ruthless perverts or as powerless "victims".[67] This will involve the development of a creative symbolic politics, which can translate complex issues into immediately comprehensible images with which audiences can easily identify their own social experience of frustration with bureaucracy, "the cuts", party politics, and so on. This is especially important, since any question of the real pressing needs of people with HIV infection and disease are so often dismissed as special pleading, or as calls for "positive discrimination" at other people's expense. We therefore have to make it clear that the issue of health care provision is one that far exceeds the treatment of HIV, and that the need to expand community nursing facilities and social service provision is of benefit to all. Besides, arguments that contrast the cost of treatment drugs for people with HIV to, say, the fact that local authorities are counting the knives and forks in old people's homes, invariably draw on a lightly veiled version of mainstream AIDS ideology which effectively advocates straightforward triage as the only long-term solution to the problems of community health care provision. Indeed, it is precisely the depravity of a social order that can calmly justify the denial of adequate life-saving resources to one social group in favour of another that the politics of AIDS exposes with shocking clarity.

In this respect we can learn a great deal from the example of ACT UP, which organizes regular "die-ins" at political and medical conferences, and in other culturally symbolic "public" spaces, where hundreds of people lie down on the ground to represent the otherwise invisible dead, with messages on their T-shirts which read: "Dead From Red Tape", "Bush Victim", and so on. In a similar manner rows of ACT UP demonstrators stand up at meetings to interrupt complacent politicians and health officials, waving their wrist-watches set to the alarm position above their heads, chanting: "We don't have time! We don't have time!" We need to learn to use public events like the birth of a royal baby in a private hospital as a media stage for our issues, in order to contrast the situation of mothers and babies with HIV in NHS care, in front of the inevitable waiting cameras. We have to be able to fill the churches of bigoted anti-gay clergy with lesbians and gay men, as the British Gay Christian Movement did in 1988. We have to be able to read off the profit margins of the pharmaceutical industry against the HIV statistics on the steps of the Stock Exchange and outside Downing Street on Budget Day. We need a politics of representation that can expose the real consequences of familial ideology, and its impoverished vision of what it means to be a woman or a man, a parent or a child in contemporary Britain. The fashionable "market forces" picture of human health and sexuality insists that people with HIV "choose" to get ill, and that gay men "choose" homosexuality. The "answer" in this view is simply to deny anyone the right to "choose" to be gay, thereby defending both "the family" and "public health", which are thus conveniently more closely aligned than ever. Yet the same view tragically fails to recognize the reality of heterosexual HIV transmission, and is obliged to regard heterosexuals with HIV as "special cases", homosexualized as it were by their diagnosis.[68] It is the brutal banality of this world view that our politics has to be able to lay bare.

The examples of the lesbian activists who climbed down ropes into the House of Lords during the Section 28 debates, and the women who broke into a BBC news broadcast to protest against this discriminatory legislation, demonstrate the ways in which an effective political theatre of images can begin to be constructed, seducing the ever voyeuristic mass media, invading "public" spaces in order to challenge the "official" cultural agenda of AIDS. As Stuart Hall points out: "In this day and age, in our kind of society, politics is either conducted *ideologically* or not at all."[69] The cultural politics of AIDS stands at the intersection of many different histories — of medicine, gay liberation, feminism, the pharmaceutical industry, the press, the criminalization of injecting drug use, racism, and so on. It is up to us to establish the threads connecting these different sites of struggle and contestation, especially in relation to the overarching question of health care provision and health promotion. These need not be dull and uninspiring words, reeking of an antiseptic politics of welfarism, and "do-gooding". Our greatest challenge is to be able to construct a politics of health that can speak across the barriers of class and race and gender and sexuality, providing a powerful collective vision of how our lives could be. As David Hockney put it so aptly in a recent interview: "We're all frail, you know. You make the best you can of life, you know. And they won't acknowledge that. They cannot see how people try and live their lives with some love in it."[70]

One of the great triumphs of Thatcherism has been to tap in successfully to people's sense of vulnerability. But vulnerability to what? As Raymond Williams wrote not long before his death: "What matters, always, is the way production is organized ... It is also, and now crucially, the way in which priorities between *different forms of production* are decided."[71] We are systematically poisoned by the food we eat, the air we breathe, the very seas and rivers we bathe in and the water we drink. The whole question of the quality of our lives is up for grabs, including the dreadfully impoverished models for human social and sexual relationships that so dominate Western culture. There is no point in our timidly wishing to be readmitted to "the family" on the terms in which it has been ideologically established. For it is precisely "the family" that lies at the heart of so many of our society's most grievous psychic injuries and injustices. One major aspect of the challenge of a radical politics of health must involve the re-imagining of how human relations might be.

This in turn draws us back to the question of "communities" and communitarian values. Community remains a word which is "still used to sugar all kinds of top-down interventions".[72] In one powerful Thatcherite sense it remains intransigently hostile to any notions of social or cultural diversity, an embattled fortress of "traditional values". For many socialists it is the embodiment of liberalism, undermining "class solidarity". AIDS commentary speaks frequently of "community care" with an approving tone, assuming that the communities it describes are precise localities, actual places, rather than loose networks of diverse, contingent interests, identities, and values. There is thus an inevitable tension between the state's emphasis on voluntary community care, and the people actually involved in caring. Contrary to much popular opinion, there has never been a strong sense of gay community in Britain. This is hardly surprising when one considers the extraordinary cultural and sexual conservatism of British society, most clearly expressed in its age of consent laws. Yet HIV has brought into being a community of interests which includes doctors, nurses, parents, friends, and all those caught up with the grim routine of a tragedy which is still widely regarded as a just retribution. It is from this unity that we can build new alliances, create new identities, make new friends, always remembering that: "In a permanently transitional age we must *expect* unevenness, contradictory outcomes, disjunctures, delays, contingencies, uncompleted projects, overlapping emergent ones."[73]

Stuart Hall has described just such a politics of health, one aspect of the larger "struggle for popular identities", a politics that: "must draw to itself the widest range of popular aspirations about health and enable different sorts of people to see themselves reflected in this emerging conception of health and thus come increasingly to identify with it."[74] This means in practice that we have to begin from the most fundamental acknowledgement of all, our shared mortality, and our inevitable susceptibility to sickness and disease. Those of us who think of ourselves as "well", live our lives under the shadow of an immense forgetfulness. For we have all been ill, and will be ill again. We are also living with a culturally institutionalized failure of historical memory, concerning the situation that prevailed in Britain before the creation of the National Health Service, and the emergence of what one American writer has described as: "the current epidemic of sexual piety."[75] At the same time we can never draw sufficient attention to the degrading treatment of the disabled, the elderly, the homeless and the insane in contemporary Britain, all suffering the direct predictable consequence of "free choice", market dominated capitalism, and its radical incompatibility with effective and adequately financed national health care provision in the public sector. Hence the immediate significance of the emergent Community Research Initiative (CRI) movement, described else-where in this book by Meurig Horton, as a profoundly innovative alternative to existing practices of medical research and treatment. Our aim is to empower people collectively, to encourage them to identify and reject with confidence the ideology of AIDS. This involves profound questions concerning our relations to sources of "information" and their authority. In one of his most moving and stimulating asides, the late Michel Foucault asked: "What would be the value of the passion for knowledge if it resulted only in a certain amount of knowledgeableness and not, in one way or another and to the extent possible, in the knower's straying afield of himself? There are times in life when the question of knowing if one can think differently than one thinks, and perceive differently than one sees, is absolutely necessary if one is to go on looking and reflecting at all."[76] The world-wide scale of HIV infection and disease, and their long-term consequences, only serve to underscore the significance of his intellectual commitment to laying bare the workings of power, not only at its most nakedly brutal and oppressive points, but in its most intimate and elusive aspects. Dr Allan Brandt points out that, "Diseases are complex bio-ecological problems that may be mitigated only by addressing a range of scientific, social and political considerations. No single intervention — even an effective

8. Joanne Aronson Burges & Donna Slotin, "Families In Touch : Understanding AIDS", *The Chicago Tribune*, November 1988.

9. Stuart Hall, *The Hard Road To Renewal : Thatcherism and the Crisis of the Left*, London 1988, p. 8.

10 Simon Watney, "The Day After Hiroshima : Some Reflections on Official British and Swedish AIDS Education Materials and Government Policies", Stockholm 1988.

11. David Brindle, "Row over vetting of AIDS manual", *The Guardian*, Thursday, 22 September 1988, p. 3; and, Annabel Ferriman, "Officials stop new AIDS pack", *The Observer*, Sunday, 2 October 1988, p. 8.

12. World Summit of Ministers of Health, London Declaration On AIDS Prevention, 28 January 1988, Declaration no. 6 : "We emphasize the need in AIDS prevention programmes to protect human rights and human dignity. Discrimination against, and stigmatization of, HIV infected people and people with AIDS undermine public health and must be avoided."

13. see Simon Watney, *Policing Desire : Pornography, AIDS and the Media*, London 1987, chapter 4.

14. Jeffrey Weeks, *Sexuality*, London 1986, p. 81.

15. "Thatcher mocks right to be gay," *Capital Gay*, no. 314, 16 October 1987.

16. "Thatcher claims Wesley as ally," *The Guardian*, Thursday, 26 May 1988, p. 2.

17. Nicholas de Jongh, "Thatcher 'pushed to keep Clause 28'", *The Guardian*, Friday, 8 April 1988, p. 1.

18. Douglas Keay, "AIDS, Education And The Year 2000", *Woman's Own*, 31 October 1987, p. 10.

19. Michel Foucault, "On Governmentality", *Ideology & Consciousness* no. 6, 1979.

20. Dr Joan M. Woodley, "AIDS concern misplaced", *General Practitioner*, 6 March 1987, p. 16.

21. Dr T. Russell, "Gay acts are immoral", *General Practitioner*, 18 March 1988, p. 18. (I would like to thank Dr Simon Mansfield for drawing my attention to this and the previous reference.)

22. Raymond Williams, "Democracy and Parliament", *Marxism Today*, June 1982, p. 17.

23. ibid., p. 18.

24. David Edgar, op. cit.

25. see Richard Plant, *The Pink Triangle: The Nazi War Against Homosexuals*, Edinburgh 1987, p. 110.

26. A phrase used several times during the Prime Minister's closing speech at the annual Conservative Party Conference in Brighton, Friday, 14 October 1988.

27. see Peter Aggleton & Hilary Homans, "Health Education, HIV Infection & AIDS", in Aggleton & Homans (eds.), *Social Aspects of AIDS*, London 1988.

28. Dr A. R. Moss, "Predicting who will progress to AIDS", *British Medical Journal*, vol. 297, Saturday, 29 October 1988.

29. Dr June E. Osborn, "AIDS: Politics And Science", *The New England Journal Of Medicine*, 18 February 1988, p. 445.

30. ibid.

31. Claudine Herzlich & Janine Perret, "Illness : From Causes To Meaning", in Caroline Currer & Margaret Stacey (eds.), *Concepts Of Health And Disease : A Comparative Perspective*, Leamington Spa, 1986, p. 75.

32. Honourable exceptions have been the work of Duncan Campbell in *New Statesman & Society*, and the work of James Erlichman and David Worsfold in *The Guardian.*

33. Clare Dover, "Britain's £1bn AIDS bill", *Daily Express*, Friday, 2 December 1988, p. 19.

34. Graham Turner, "Is There A Homosexual Conspiracy?", *The Sunday Telegraph*, 5 June 1988, p. 17.

35. "Vice squad rejects 'crude' AIDS leaflet", *The Guardian*, 15 April 1988.

36. Paul Smith and Graham Dudman "Blaze Heroes In AIDS Scare", *Daily Mail*, Saturday, 21 November 1987, p. 1. For a more recent example of this type of story see Mark Christy, "Crash Hero's AIDS Peril", *Daily Star*, Wednesday, 28 December 1988, p. 1.

37. Simon Watney, *Policing Desire*, p. 137.

38. see Simon Watney, "AIDS, Language and The Third World" elsewhere in this book.

39. see Cindy Patton, "Inventing African AIDS", *City Limits* no. 363, 15–22 September 1988, p. 85; and Simon Watney, "Missionary Positions: AIDS 'Africa' & Race", *Differences: A Journal Of Feminist Cultural Studies*, no. 1, 1989.

40. see Simon Watney, "The Spectacle Of AIDS", *October* no. 43, winter 1987, reprinted in Douglas Crimp (ed.), *AIDS: Cultural Analysis/Cultural Activism*, Cambridge, MA 1988.

41. ibid.

42. see Simon Watney, "Our Rights And Our Dignity", *Gay Times* issue 114, March 1988.

43. e.g. Paul Monnette, *Borrowed Time : An AIDS Memoir*, London 1988, p. 1.

44. Simon Watney, *Policing Desire*, chapter 3. See also Paula Treichler, "AIDS, homophobia and biomedical discourse : an epidemic of signification", *Cultural Studies* vol. 1, no. 3, October 1987.

45. see Simon Watney, "Desperate Straits", *Gay Times* issue 116, May 1988, p. 12.

46. Clare Dover, " 'Straight sex' thousands are infected with AIDS", *Daily Express*, Tuesday, 1 November 1988, p. 5.

47. see Robert R. Redfield & Donald S. Burke, "HIV Infection : The Clinical Picture", *Scientific American*, vol. 259 no. 4, October 1988.

48. see Cindy Patton, *Sex and Germs : The Politics Of AIDS*, Boston, MA 1985; also Brian A. Evans et al, "Trends in sexual behaviour and risk factors for HIV infection among homosexual men, 1984–87", *British Medical Journal*, vol. 298, 28 January 1989.

49. e.g. in Britain "Memorandum by the Conservative Family Campaign to the 1987 Social Services Committee", Minutes of Evidence, London 1988; or Dr Goodson-Wickes, House of Commons, *Hansard*, 17 February 1988, asking "the Chancellor of the Duchy of Lancaster if he will take steps to cease the distribution by the citizens' advice bureau in Wimbledon of the pamphlet *Sex*, published by the Terrence Higgins Trust, in view of its explicit promotion of exclusively homosexual activities." In the United States, see the Helms Amendment, *Congressional Record — Senate*, 14 October, 1987.

50. see Kaye Wellings, "Heterosexual spread of AIDS : a challenge for health education", *Health Education Journal*, vol. 46, no. 4, 1987.

51. *AIDS-UK*, issue 3, November 1988, Health Education Authority, p. 1.

52. In June 1988, a total of 1,464 injecting drug users with HIV had been recorded in Britain, and 54 with AIDS: *AIDS-UK*, issue 3, November 1988.

53. see Dr A. R. Moss, op. cit. See also "The Helquist Report", *The Advocate*, issue 512, 22 November 1988.

54. Sir Alfred Sherman, "AIDS Charter rebuff", *The Times*, Wednesday, 14 December 1988, p. 17.

55. Aileen Bailantyne, "AIDS drive had little impact", *The Guardian*, Thursday, 29 September 1988, p. 7.

56. Sherman, op. cit.

57. reprinted in Michael Callen, (ed.) *Surviving And Thriving With AIDS*, PWA Coalition, New York 1987.

58. see Simon Watney, "The Wrong Ideas That Are Plaguing AIDS", *The Guardian*, Friday, 16 October 1987, p. 22.

59. Philip M. Boffey, "Campaign To Find Drugs For Fighting AIDS Is Intensified", *The New York Times*, Monday, 15 February 1988, p. A14.

60. I am grateful to Meurig Horton for this point.

61. see Simon Watney, "Acting Up", *Square Peg*, no. 21, 1988; also Sarah Payton, "ACT UP", *Spare Rib*, no. 197, December 1988/January 1989.

62. Douglas Crimp, "Introduction", in Crimp (ed.) *AIDS : Cultural Analysis Cultural Activism*, Cambridge, MA 1988.

63. see Greg Bordowitz. "Picture A Coalition", in Crimp op. cit.

64. The regular opening words at the weekly New York meetings of ACT UP.

65. "Ghettos? A Good Idea", editorial, *Daily Star*, 2 December 1988.

66. Nadezhda Mandelstam, *Hope Against Hope*, London 1979, p. 127.

67. The best introduction to these issues remains Stuart Hall, "The Determinations Of New Photographs", *Cultural Studies* no. 3, University of Birmingham Centre For Contemporary Cultural Studies, autumn 1977.

68. see Cindy Patton, "Safer Sex and Lesbians", *The Pink Paper*, issue 14, 25 February 1988, p. 2.

69. Stuart Hall, "Thatcher's Lessons", *Marxism Today*, March 1988, p. 23.

70. Simon Watney, "Portrait Of An Artist", *Marxism Today*, October 1988, p. 45.

71. Raymond Williams, *Socialism And Ecology*, London 1982, p. 15.

72. N. J. Derrincourt, "Strategies of Community Care", in Martin Loney, et. al. (eds.) *Social Policy & Social Welfare*, Milton Keynes 1983, p. 271.

73. Stuart Hall, "Brave New World", *Marxism Today*, October 1988, p. 24.

74. Stuart Hall, *The Hard Road to Renewal*, p. 282.

75. Susan Jacoby, "Risky Business", *The New York Times*, Section 6, Sunday, 24 April 1988, p. 26.

76. Michel Foucault, *The History Of Sexuality Volume 2 : The Uses Of Pleasure*, London 1987, p. 8.

77. Dr Allan M. Brandt, "AIDS In Historical Perspective : Four Lessons from the History of Sexually Transmitted Diseases", *American Journal of Public Health*, vol. 78, no. 4, April 1988, p. 371.

78. Cindy Patton, "Safer Sex and Lesbians", op. cit.

79. James Baldwin, *The Fire Next Time*, p. 124.

80. Antonio Gramsci, "The Formation of Intellectuals", in *The Modern Prince & other Writings*, New York 1967, p. 122.

The advertisement is marked by the same contradiction that has been the hallmark of official media campaigns to combat AIDS in Britain. On the one hand, the British public is charged to equip itself with the facts of AIDS and HIV infection: "Don't Die of Ignorance," says the billboard caption. But equally powerfully conveyed by this television advertisement's use of stock narrative and visual conventions — the AIDS sufferer as mute victim and vision of horror, the body positive as a man condemned — is the danger of identification with those affected by HIV or AIDS. The hospital narrative represents the dividing-line between the sick and the healthy as immutable. Once the hospital visitor becomes a patient, he is as good as dead; now we recognize ourselves in him at our peril.

In the wake of the first nationwide media campaign on AIDS and HIV infection, twenty speakers and an audience of one hundred and sixty met at the Institute of Contemporary Arts (ICA), London, for a conference we called "AIDS: the Cultural Agenda". Our aim as organizers — myself and Katy Sender from the ICA, Simon Watney as outside consultant — was to bring together AIDS activists and public health workers from Britain and the United States with representatives of the cultural-theoretical avant-garde who were the ICA's traditional constituency. To that latter group, the message of official media campaigns should, in theory at least, have been anathema. On billboards and television screens across the country, AIDS was being visualized as an abitrary configuration of signifiers of horror: slate-blue tombstones rising out of swirling dry ice, menacing background music, the ubiquitous invocation, "Don't Die of Ignorance." The campaign was widely criticized at the time for its failure to provide basic information on the nature of HIV infection or its distinction from ARC and AIDS, and the risk of transmission through unsafe sex, needle sharing, or in pregnancy. While raising public awareness of AIDS as a threat to the nation, it offered scant resolution to these newly awakened public anxieties. As Judith Williamson points out in her article in this collection, AIDS, and by association those suffering from the disease, has been made a metaphor for what the French psychoanalyst Julia Kristeva terms "the abject": the psychic domain of unnamed horror, terror and loss of selfhood. Thus, in the first nationwide campaign against AIDS in Britain, AIDS was harnessed as a convenient keyword for a general social threat to an undifferentiated population: "It can kill anyone," (billboard caption). Alongside other forms of social deviance and physical disintegration (viz. other government campaigns against heroin and drunk driving), images of AIDS were slotted into an official rhetoric of public insecurity, in which the sick, the poor and the deviant figured as threats to the prevailing social and moral order. An infantilized population — defined as healthy, but "ignorant" — was called upon to trust information from a government committed to the maintenance of a puritan and socially divisive order. As the London listings magazine *City Limits* put it at the time: "Alongside heroin and other 'social issue' campaigns, the Government, entrenched in its unpopularity, can be seen to be doing 'something' for the public good. In addition, (AIDS) has added grist to the Tory 'family values' campaign. [Junior] Health Minister Edwina Currie and Mary Whitehouse were in the front line espousing the virtues of marriage and monogamy . . . Meanwhile, the issue of safe sex and how to practice it has taken a back seat . . ."[3]

By 1987, then, the British government had set a very clear cultural agenda in relation to HIV which, sadly, did not always coincide with effective AIDS prevention, care or cure. At a time when fewer than a thousand cases of AIDS had been reported in this country, popular experience of the syndrome — except in the communities directly affected — was minimal; yet its cultural impact, through film, advertising, leaflet and billboard campaigns, was phenomenal.

Barely in evidence, by contrast, were critical cultural responses to the crisis and its official handling. In the official education campaign, the British public was offered one of two mutually opposed social identities: it could align itself with the healthy populace at large, or it had perforce to take the position of the victim of HIV infection or AIDS who, as Simon Watney has pointed out,[4] is repeatedly constructed as the source, not the sufferer of the mortal threat posed by the epidemic.

That fixing of identity should have laid the campaign open to widespread criticism from cultural analysts, who had argued for two decades at least that stable identity is a chimera, and disease a construction of language and social practice. What the literary critic Jonathan Dollimore has called "materialist accounts of deviance"[5] (and he refers primarily, though not exclusively, to the work of Michel Foucault) have shown how social institutions — or more precisely, the languages and practices that inhabit them — mark out categories of "otherness" to be occupied by the sick, the aberrant, the socially deviant. From this, we should have learned that the identity of AIDS victim, with its associations of social and sexual deviance has to be analysed — and combated — as the product of a repressive rhetoric of medical and social regulation. Certainly, that contention has been explored, most centrally in this country by Simon Watney in his book *Policing Desire*, and in passing in other contexts. Thus Frank Mort, in his history of medical and moral politics since the nineteenth century, *Dangerous Sexualities*, refers briefly to AIDS as "the contemporary moment in a much longer history, the extraordinarily complex interweaving of medicine and morality with the surveillance and regulation —even the very defintion — of sex. The disease has produced gay men as its victims, and their sexuality as the problem. This is part of the norms, protocols and procedures written into the history of medico-moral discourse."[6] Those themes — the use of AIDS as a regulatory force, its implications for social and sexual identities — had been taken up, too, in journalistic pieces published in the left and feminist press prior to the ICA conference by many of the participants.[7] Such responses, however, remained sparse and scattered, isolated on the one hand from wider public debates on a universally feared pandemic, and largely divorced from the activism of affected communities.

What in this context could be the possible contribution of an institution such as the ICA? To answer that question will require a brief detour through the history of the ICA as a major institution of the British avant-garde. That history in turn will raise two issues: the question of the part to be played by cultural theorists and critics in generating effective responses to AIDS; and that of the role of national arts institutions, the ICA among them, in combating social crisis on the scale of the AIDS epidemic.

The Avant-Garde Legacy
In his book *The End of Art Theory*, the visual artist and theorist Victor Burgin makes passing reference to a conference staged at the ICA many years prior to the 1988 AIDS conference. Entitled "The State of British Art", this 1977 event purported to offer a response to what it claimed was a "crisis" in British art. But, as Burgin wryly observes: "I never did learn what the 'crisis' in British art was; nor, I suspect, did anyone else. In retrospect, some ten years on, I now see the ICA

event, the brainchild of three British art critics, as a textbook example of what psychoanalysis terms projection: the crisis sensed by these critics was not in art but in criticism itself."[8]

For Burgin, then, this rhetoric of crisis signals a sea change in the history of British criticism, not only in the fine arts (indeed here, that change took place much later than in other disciplines, film and photography in particular), but across the wider field of cultural critique. Distinguishing criticism by its operation within "common sense" — as opposed to theory, which questions common sense in order to replace it, where necessary, with "better-founded, or more comprehensive explanations"[9] — he traces the intellectual and political developments which inaugurated a "crisis in the very culture in whose name criticism pronounced its judgments":

> Political dissent was not the only French import of the late 1960s and the 1970s, there was also a massive influx of theory. Introduced into Britain by *New Left Review*, and then developed in a variety of other journals, most notably . . . *Screen*, French marxism, semiotics and psychoanalysis became the radical alternatives to the discourse of Art in general, and the empirical-intuitive Anglo-Saxon critical tradition in particular."[10]

What Victor Burgin describes in *The End of Art Theory* is a process of intellectual migration — the flight of socially and politically committed artists and intellectuals away from established cultural institutions, and into the marginal arena of critical cultural practice and political activism — which had profound significance for the ICA. Since its foundation in 1947, the ICA had identified itself closely with the vanguard of European modernism. Its first exhibition paid homage to "Forty Years of Modern Art": British artists such as Bacon, Moore and Sutherland featured alongside Braque, Chagall, Ernst, Magritte, Kandinsky, Picasso. That vanguardist tradition has since been jealously guarded. When the ICA moved from its first premises in Dover Street to its current location in The Mall, its founders iconoclastically proclaimed, "The Ivory Tower has been demolished." And in the ICA's 1987 fortieth anniversary booklet, that comment is cited as fully in keeping with the "spirit of independence" that remains the moving force behind the institution today.

In thus reiterating its allegiance to the modernist impulse out of which it was founded, the ICA, however, has posed itself a dilemma. Will its affiliation in future be to the tradition of high modernism, with its classic distancing of "art" from "life", of aesthetic experience from social and political realities? That conservative tradition is certainly reasserting itself in the British arts in the eighties: witness for example the 1988 launch by art critic Peter Fuller of the high-gloss magazine *Modern Painters* which, true to its title (its predecessor was Ruskin's nineteenth-century journal of the same name), attempts to revitalize an aesthetic philosophy that stresses the permanent and timeless aspects of modern art and its separation from practical experience. Or will the ICA instead retrieve from modernism the legacy of what US critic Andreas Huyssen calls the "historical avant-garde" — of "that art which more than any other challenged the values and traditions of bourgeois culture"[11] — an art unique in the strength of its social and political engagement?

The dilemma discerned by Victor Burgin, looking back to the 1977 "State of British Art" conference, is, then, one that does not only concern the institution of criticism; it has dogged the ICA itself throughout its post-war history. At this moment in the late seventies, the separation Burgin notes between "criticism" and "theory" was mirrored by a rift between arts institutions and the oppositional publics that had emerged from the movements of '68 and after. In the ensuing decade, however, the contemporary art world has seen the rise to dominance of the ensemble of artistic and intellectual practices we now call "postmodernism".

Postmodernism, as formulated within art criticism, has been identified with a set of techniques and strategies amongst which Michael Newman, in his "critical lexicon" of postmodernism, lists the denial of authorship, the use of allegory, bricolage, parody and simulation.[12] But most centrally for our purposes, there has been what Andreas Huyssen calls a "major shift of . . . interest from, the early two-pronged concern (of the avant-garde) with popular culture and experimental art and theory to a new focus on cultural theory."[13] Under the guise of postmodernism, theory has once again made a home for itself in the established institutions of contemporary art in Britain.

The ICA has played a major part in instituting that shift in British artistic and intellectual practice. Many of the artists shown at the ICA through the 1980s (the names are numerous, but they might include Cindy Sherman, Mary Kelly, Robert Mapplethorpe, Imants Tillers) work self-consciously within the frame of reference of a politicized theory whose project is to unsettle prevailing assumptions about language and culture. Barbara Kruger, whose work features on the cover of *Taking Liberties*, was described when she showed at the ICA in 1983 as creating "jarring linguistic and visual equations" which "displace language and disorient the law." Such a blossoming of theoretical interest has been reflected, too, in the ICA Talks programme which, through the 1980s, has played an active part in the British appropriation of continental cultural and psychoanalytic theory. By 1984, the ICA had launched a publications series, ICA Documents, which, on the basis of ICA seminars and conferences, explored psychoanalytic, French structuralist and poststructuralist theory, through papers by and discussions with key intellectual figures– among them Julia Kristeva, Jacques Derrida, Jean-François Lyotard, to name but the most prominent. Alongside the new generation of cultural-theoretical journals — *Theory, Culture and Society, New Formations, ZG,* or art-form specific publications such as *Block, Screen* and *Ten 8* — the ICA Documents series helped put into circulation ideas that are central to the critical analysis of postmodernism and postmodernity: notions of the fragmentation of identities, of the dispersed nature of power, of the significance of deconstruction as critical strategy.

"Theory," however, is an ambiguous instrument with which to engage contemporary cultural realities. Publicly and in muttered private expressions of grievance, the work represented at the ICA has been criticized as difficult and inaccessible, the institution itself as elitist and isolationist. So for example the former art critic and now literary editor of the liberal daily *The Guardian* — who has in the past often been fulsome in his support of ICA work — responded to the ICA's fortieth anniversary fund-raising appeal with an article which opens: "From centre for creative protest the ICA has become a playground for a declining civilization". Waldemar Januszczak continues:

> The ICA . . . was, by all accounts, born of a cosy private members club set up by disillusioned intellectuals for disillusioned intellectuals — a place to share the pursuit of civilization with a like-minded few. It is an attitude which has persisted, and indeed seems to be making a guilt-free comeback in the Thatcher years . . . The ICA has been comprehensively depoliticized. It has grown up into a trough for trendies.[14]

Trendy or not, the audience drawn to theoretical debates at the ICA today certainly no longer occupies the political positions of the early seventies (though whether this qualifies as "depoliticization" is questionable). Through the 1980s, the oppositional movements which Burgin saw as the seedbed for seventies critical theory are increasingly marginalized and fragmented. In that context, the cultural-political function of the ICA has indeed changed. No longer servicing an already constituted critical community, it must either content itself with packaging theory for the discrete "audience segments" of the contemporary art-world-as-market — Baudrillardian postmodernism for the glitterati, mother-child psychoanalysis for the worried mothers of post-feminism. Alternatively, it can work to forge new connections between "theory" and the praxis of emerging oppositional constituencies. This, precisely, was what motivated the 1988 conference on AIDS. Until that date, the theoretical avant-garde had remained largely silent on the subject of AIDS. When Simon Watney first approached the ICA in 1986 to run a conference we initially titled "AIDS culture", he was able to name writers and possible speakers — a handful in Britain, many more in the US — who were bringing the social and cultural theories energetically debated at the ICA to bear on an activist politics of AIDS. We saw here the potential to wrest from avant-garde cultural theory the "precious heritage of . . . materials, practices and strategies"[15] it bequeathes to a contemporary cultural politics. We said "yes" to the conference.

Art Against AIDS in Britain?

The rest is the history of which this book is a document. The conference was finally staged eighteen months after the first planning meeting. Running over two days, it brought together diverse constituencies of cultural workers — media workers and analysts with AIDS activists, social and cultural theorists with professional health workers — to debate the cultural dimensions of the epidemic in the US and Britain. At a time when official media campaigns were representing those affected by AIDS and HIV infection as the source of a threat to security of the nation; at a time when AIDS threatened to be used to legitimate official strategies of social control and sexual policing, the ICA conference aimed to contribute to the efforts of affected communities to shift and refocus public debate on AIDS.

Such efforts to intervene in the field of public representations of AIDS will continually be subject to strategies of marginalization. On one level, the prevailing common sense about AIDS and HIV infection — that they are best dealt with exclusively by medical experts — will be used to screen out from public consciousness artistic and cultural responses to the epidemic. That point was amply demonstrated by press coverage of the ICA conference; as the world's press assembled for the World Health Organization conference at the Barbican, the ICA press conference was attended by a small handful of journalists, most with a track record in lesbian and gay coverage. The paucity of post-conference press responses — there was national coverage only in the lesbian and gay press, and one piece in *City Limits* — not only indicated the extent to which the cultural politics of AIDS continues to be marginalized as a "gay issue". It was indicative, too, of the degree to which access to participation in public debate on AIDS is restricted in this country. Since the Health Education Authority was designated as the body with responsibility for education nationwide on AIDS, the production and dissemination of representations of AIDS and HIV infection have been massively regulated by central government. The HEA itself is directly subject to the Health Department under minister Kenneth Clarke. Its educational programmes are centrally vetted, and censored: one entire education pack for schools was withdrawn on the grounds of its failure to promote family values. In that context, arts institutions could in future offer precious resources for the production of alternative, critical cultural forms. Whether they will do so depends on their ability to sustain a sense of their practical, social function: a commitment to what one of the ICA's founders, Herbert Read, called "art in its social origins . . . oriented towards the future".[16]

Notes

1. B. Ruby Rich, "Only Human: Sex, Gender and Other Misrepresentations", in 1987 American Film Institute Video Festival, Los Angeles 1987, p. 42.
2. Douglas Crimp, "AIDS: Cultural Analysis/Cultural Activism", in *October*, no. 43, 1987, p. 15.
3. Kathy Myers, "AIDS: The Sale of Safe Sex", in *City Limits*, 11 December 1987, p. 17.

JUDITH WILLIAMSON

EVERY VIRUS TELLS A STORY

The Meanings of HIV and AIDS

Nothing could be more meaningless than a virus. It has no point, no purpose, no plan; it is part of no scheme, carries no inherent significance. And yet nothing is harder for us to confront than the complete absence of meaning. By its very definition, meaninglessness cannot be articulated within our social language, which is a system *of* meaning: impossible to include, as an absence, it is also impossible to exclude — for meaninglessness isn't just the opposite of meaning, it is the end of meaning and threatens the fragile structures by which we make sense of the world.

What has this to do with AIDS? As the intentionless HIV virus enters our highly coded culture, saturated as it is with teleological structures, narratives that seem to be going somewhere, that impossible conflict between meaninglessness and meaning can go in two directions which are not alternatives but feed off each other and oscillate endlessly. Both have a profound effect on the way in which our society represents and perceives AIDS — and, more specifically, the HIV virus, whose attack on the immune system results in the conditions that characterize the syndrome.

In one version, the virus becomes endowed with the purpose it lacks: at its crudest, this can be seen in the retribution theories peddled by Moral Majority figures like Jerry Falwell, who claims that God sent AIDS as a punishment to homosexuals (though babies and haemophiliacs pose more of a problem). But while it is relatively easy to counter hysterical conservatism, it is less easy to pin down the wider sense in which AIDS takes its place within the narrative systems along whose tracks events seem to glide quite naturally, whether in news reports, movie plots or everyday explanations. But even as AIDS is invested with meaning through these structures, that meaninglessness which is thereby negated lurks ominously at the edges of perception, at once a threat, and a constant spur, to the formation of explanatory fictions.

Of course, there are many things besides the HIV virus which threaten established patterns of thinking. In particular, sex and death are always liable to tear through that familiar fabric which clothes our naked experience — yet these are precisely the events that are most highly coded, most central to so many fictions. They are also inevitably linked with AIDS: sex as a means of HIV transmission, death as its probable outcome. It is no coincidence that sex and death are events of the body: the point at which we meet, and are a part of, the material world, no longer imposers of meaning on it but imposed upon by its meaninglessness.

Homosexuality, too, which threatens the socially endorsed structure of the family (also a narrative: grow up, get married, have children, repeat . . .) is inextricably linked with first-world perceptions of AIDS and HIV. So one way and another the AIDS discourse of our society is structured and coded precisely to fend off transgression, or what Julia Kristeva has called "the weight of meaninglessness", the *abject* which cannot be contemplated except as something to be ejected from the self.

My argument, then, is that in the dominant perceptions of HIV/AIDS in our culture two (related) things happen. On the one hand, the HIV virus enters a kind of Noddy-land of narrative meaning, where it takes on particular characteristics, goals and functions — even "preferences". On the other, however, it joins the morass of unthinkability in which homosexuality is already (for many people) placed, a Gothic territory where fears are flung out into a sort of mental wasteland beyond the castle walls of the ego. In the first part of this essay I want to look at the busy-bee virus in its purposeful mode as dramatized within various fictions; in the second, I will return to the notion of the "abject" and look not at the purposeful, but its opposite, the imagery of disintegration which resists this narrativization, even while emanating from it.

After teaching and writing about films for many years I am convinced that the structures we call "genres" within fiction are not restricted to movies and novels but also characterize the "structures of feeling", to borrow Raymond Williams's phrase, of our everyday life. If a genre can broadly be defined as a pattern of narrative and imagery, then the patterns of almost all film genres can be found in press reporting, ordinary conversation, general perceptions of political and personal events. Narrative structures are enormously important to our way of thinking: we like things to have a beginning, a middle and an end, we like events to have a point, to seem to be going somewhere. *Closure* is the word used in literary criticism to describe this finished, purposeful feel of fictional narratives. And, of course, fictional structures *are* purposeful — nothing happens by chance in a book or film, every detail is there to further the story in some way.

So genres are groups of narratives that share a particular structure of concerns and characteristics, and involve particular sets of images. The two that I want to argue are most mobilized around AIDS are Horror and Melodrama. Horror in films is closely linked to the Gothic in novels, that genre which was so popular in the eighteenth and nineteenth centuries, where demons and monsters threaten the innocent, and nature — including human nature — is constantly fearsome. The other modern genre of film and television which is constantly employed in "sympathetic" understandings of AIDS is melodrama — a form whose sentimentality is in many ways the flip side of Horror's brutality. Historically, both the Gothic and the Sentimental were strands within Romanticism: a mode which above all else heroizes the individual and — as is evident in so many well-known Romantic poems — seeks a purpose in Nature. Cut off from society, the individual is located within a natural world which may threaten (in Gothic terms) or embrace (in Sentimental) him (and it usually is him); but this natural world is never neutral.

There is a further genre which is often associated with the writing and understanding of AIDS, and may also appear as an antidote or counter-plot in horror or melodrama, and that is the detective story. A search for sources is a large part of the teleological or goal-directed mode of thinking which characterizes both rationalist/modernist thought, and, of course, all fictional narratives — which, being finished constructs, always *do* have a predetermined goal. But the classic horror film, for example, involves a search for specialist forms of knowledge: in most vampire films, a Goodie has at some stage to find an ancient, leather-bound volume which explains how to put a stake through the heart of a vampire and usefully mentions that demons can't stand garlic or the sign of the cross. More recent forms of Horror also involve specialist knowledge, for example, that zombies don't like fire. These horror-knowledge antidotes are no more daft than some of the things people think will protect them against AIDS. The relevant point here is that in thinking of horror we are accustomed to expecting specialist knowledge to allow comprehension, control and, ultimately, elimination of the threat. Medical knowledge is most frequently seen in this light, as if each problem were a keyhole merely waiting for a particular key. And a central part of the knowledge that the detective/scientist must unravel is that of origins. Whodunnit?

Within Horror, the answer to this question is always the monster — whether creature from black lagoon, space invader, giant pod or whatever. The construction of the monstrous is a way of explaining all ills, rather as a child will say that Mr Nobody spilt the milk or ate the cake: it militates against the perception of the systemic nature of problems, focusing blame instead on a particular scapegoat. This phenomenon was strikingly obvious in mythologies surrounding the fire at London's Kings Cross underground station in November 1987 (in which thirty-one people died). The lengthy public inquiry into the fire revealed quite clearly that the whole structure of London Transport's senior management was at fault. Yet so hard was it to perceive the blame as a mere lack — an abdication of municipal responsibility — that it was popularly believed (an idea fostered in the tabloid press) that a mysterious arsonist was to blame for the whole tragedy. So tenacious was the wish for the disaster to have an author that, fairly late in the inquiry, people began to claim they had seen a "strange man" in overalls lurking near a trap door. His description was uncannily similar to that of Freddy Kruger, the boiler-room avenger of *Nightmare on Elm Street*.

Now, at some stage a lighted match probably did start the fire. But the idea of a crazed arsonist saves us from the unthinkably arbitrary quality of an *accident*, and makes the whole event take on a macabre sort of sense, the product of a mind, even if a deranged one. Like the Hungerford killings (where a hitherto "normal" citizen suddenly shot, at random, many of the inhabitants of this small town before committing suicide) it represents purpose gone awry. And this, I would argue, is exactly how the AIDS phenomenon appears to many people. Again, I am not talking only about the fundamentalist Right; what I am saying holds true even, for example, of a valuable campaigning account like Randy Shilts's *And the Band Played On*.

As a piece of powerful investigative journalism, this book functions in the detective vein; and yet its language is revealing and worth examining precisely because it is found within a supposedly progressive viewpoint. One of the striking aspects of the book's detective work is its espousal of the Patient Zero theory: the original HIV carrier is "irresponsible" airline steward Gaetan Dugas, portrayed as deliberately screwing and thus "deliberately" infecting as many other gay men as possible. In this narrative, as so often happens, originality is conflated with intentionality.

Gaetan has a "voracious sexual appetite": "Lovers were like suntans to him" (even his name is a bit like suntan). Like the wicked stepmother, he constantly asks his mirror if he is the fairest one of all, and this scene is repeated over and over even as he spreads contamination: "Gaetan examined himself in the mirror . . . a few more spots had had the temerity to appear on his face . . . he smiled at the thought, 'I'm still the prettiest one'." No one within Western culture can contemplate this scenario without understanding it precisely in terms of the absent Snow White (for hers is the stepmother who behaves in this way), the innocent victim of the Vain and the Bad. While Shilts's book is rationally geared to blame the entire governmental system for failing to fund research, educate the public and treat those infected, he nevertheless cannot entirely resist the wish for a source of contamination to be found, and then blamed. If Patient Zero did not exist, we would need to invent him.

The fact that the geographical source of the virus is alleged to be Africa merely feeds into the monster narratives already available to be mobilized. Shilts's language here is very telling: "Many (with AIDS) were ailing among the uncounted sick of *primitive Africa.* Slowly and almost imperceptibly, *the killer was awakening*" (my italics). This makes the virus sound exactly like a primeval monster rising from its sleep: lumbering maybe, but still a *creature.* Later in the book, Shilts describes how the city of San Francisco battled "against an encroaching viral invader," and at another point, he tells us that, "Science at last was closing in on the viral culprit that bred international death" — which sounds like the typical denouement of a B-movie Horror narrative. Elsewhere he likens the virus to terrorism (a link that much news reporting makes in reverse). What is so significant here is the *teleology* of the language, the implication that the virus is a subject — albeit a primitive one — with intentionality.

This implication is embodied in the particular grammatical construction used by most journalists in describing AIDS. It is a "killer disease" or more expansively an "unexplained killer disease". "Killer" is a noun meaning someone who kills just as a runner is someone who runs: the use of this "er" construction carries a connotation fundamentally different from, for example, those of the entirely adjectival alternatives "fatal", "deadly" or "mortal". These words would merely describe the disease: the word "killer" animates it — as if the virus tucked a Colt .45 into its belt and went out seeking its victims.

Which brings us to another fundamentally teleological construction, used, it is true, not only with AIDS but within the wider popular discourse of Horror: the idea that unintelligent substances "claim" victims. Simon Watney quotes TV presenter Christine Chapman talking about AIDS: "AIDS doesn't mind if you're gay or straight . . . and is likely to *claim more victims as time goes on.*" We are accustomed to a disaster-speak that is unable to mention the word death: "*n* lives have been lost in the ferry disaster" (as if they had simply been *mislaid*); "AIDS", however, *claims* its "victims" — as if they belonged to it! After all, you claim what's yours (baggage) or what's due to you (benefits): the verbal construction provides a narrative sense, a closure, to the whole pointless process of death, as if it were pre-ordained whom "AIDS" would "claim". This is made clearer in the particular interview quoted when the same presenter says, over a montage of faces: "You can't tell? No, *you can't tell from looking.* AIDS doesn't choose other people. AIDS can choose you."

This idea of being invisibly chosen in some predetermined way is a major part of Calvinist theology, which still underlies the world view of much Anglo-Saxon culture. Everything is, finally, part of an already ordered narrative: the less its order is actually visible, the more certain we are — by some perverse logic — that it actually exists "underneath". Notice, however, that in all this, AIDS, whether undiscriminating or picky, has become peculiarly active: "it" claims, chooses, rages, kills, with all the senseless yet directed energy of a mad axe-murderer: meanwhile those infected with HIV become peculiarly *de-*animated, "victims" waiting to be "claimed". Of course it is nothing new to object to the offensive word "victim" and some few journalists are catching on to saying "people with AIDS". Yet I also want to place this construction within its wider generic framework, the Gothic/Sentimental, in which passivity itself is mobilized to evoke terror or pity.

In the Gothic mode, passivity provides a frisson — frequently sexualized — of fear: this is most easily understood by thinking of any horror film and its mechanisms whereby the vulnerability of the victim is as important to the production of horror as is the violence of the monster. Innocent maidens lie in bed awaiting the bites of vampires. Babysitters in empty houses find that "he knows you're alone". Close to this, however, is the pity that is evoked by a similar passivity in the Sentimental mode. Things happen *to* people, in this genre, and then they *suffer*. The classic Sentimental novel elevated suffering to an art form, also to provide a frisson in the reader. So where the stress is on the *activity* of the viral monster, one might say that AIDS discourse is closest to Gothic horror, and when it is on the "passive" (non-complaining) suffering of the "victims" it moves over into Sentimentalism. Both are combined in the British government's bizarre "tombstone" campaign — a series of public health ads launched in 1986 whose imagery consisted of what appeared to be craggily Gothic icebergs turning into a marble tombstone that could have come straight from the Hammer props room, engraved with the letters "A I D S" and captioned "Don't Die of Ignorance." What the image and slogan actually invoked was threat and innocence simultaneously: a potent combination familiar to every hack nineteenth-century novelist or twentieth-century script writer. Ignorance appears as some kind of ghostly disease appropriate to a consumptive hero or heroine on the shelves of a Victorian lending library.

In his study of the sentimental novel, *Sentimentalism as Soft Romanticism*, critic R.O. Allen has called Sentimentalism "an individualism of the last resort". The appropriateness of this diagnosis to contemporary culture is evident when you consider than a paper like the *Sun* will always run a feature on, for example, a "Heartbreak Baby", but never on the reasons for the failure in, say, healthcare structures which has *produced* the "Heartbreak". Suffering becomes a commodity isolated from any systemic cause: just as the *source* of any problem can be located in Horror discourse as the Monster, equally its *effects* can be drained of any social dimension and lumped onto the individual Victim.

If I seem to be talking somewhat generally it is because I think that much of this reliance on Horror and Sentimentalism is a general trend in our culture, and it is important to separate the structure of that trend from the particularity of AIDS, which did not "cause" it, but rather, fits into those existing channels of discourse all too well. It has been particularly striking to me — given that I barely remember hearing the word used publicly during the more socially minded '50s, '60s and '70s — that the concept of *evil* seems to arise frequently today, especially in the speech of Mrs Thatcher. Whereas right and wrong are moral concepts, framed within human activity, good and evil are absolutes, cosmic values fixed beyond human control. This is too big a subject to pursue in detail in this space but the return of "evil" as a category employed by politicians shows how very close to Gothic horror our public discourse has become. Another familiar component of it is the characterization of criminals (particularly sex criminals) as "Beasts". The problem of unacceptable human behaviour is dealt with simply by locating it outside human bounds. Tabloid papers ran a "Hunt for the Beasts" in the case of a sex attack on a boy in Brighton (significantly, the term had *not* been dragged out to apply to attackers of girls, who are perceived as more "normal", i.e. heterosexual). Copywriters threw themselves with glee into the "Bid to find *monsters who attacked boy.*"

Evil monsters and beasts are part of the repertoire of horror *images*: and it is here that I want to move from looking at Horror and related genres as structures of narrative, and consider them as structures of imagery. Obviously the two are not really separate, but while the formation of narratives seems to "put things in their place", imagery can resist this process and profoundly unsettle that order. (Films are so complex and often contradictory precisely because they combine narrative *and* imagery.) As I have written elsewhere: "The horror film can eschew the logic whereby a sexual encounter may *result* in disease. Images, as Freud said, can collapse linear reasoning — the person sexually encountered *becomes* the disease." In the only narrative scenarios about AIDS our culture can manage to contemplate (and I'm talking about "sympathetic" dramas — for example on TV), unresisting gay men/the odd erring husband/prostitutes/maladjusted single women may be threatened *by* the HIV virus; but simultaneously, on another level, they represent the threat *of* the virus, and become virtually identified with it. This is one reason for examining the less obviously pernicious language of the HIV "killer" stalking its prey, for this image so easily becomes transferred to the person *carrying* the virus. Old — or I suppose I should say young — Gaetan Dugas himself is extraordinarily viral, filtering in and out of the "bloodstream" of gay sexual activity in US and Canadian bath houses. Or, returning to Africa, where the heterosexual etymology of the disease replaces homophobia with sexism and racism — the "monster" becomes predatory black prostitutes. This is the opening paragraph of an article on the "Happy Hookers of Nairobi" – found, not in the *Sun*, but on the centre pages of the *Guardian*:

> The best time to observe the Nairobi hooker is at dusk when the tropical sun dips beneath the Rift Valley and silhouettes the thorn trees against the African skyline. It is then that the hooker preens itself and emerges to stalk its prey . . . white men looking for fun and with money to burn.

The article went on to suggest that the "beast" in this case was black women's destructive sexuality: the "herds" (sic) of "prey" are, of course, drained of all responsibility.

It is a classic tenet of Horror theory that the monstrous which narrative splits off from the self is a projection of unacceptable parts of the self — and, indeed, of society. In his article "An Introduction to the American Horror Film", Robin Wood outlines his theory (drawing on Freud) of the Return of the Repressed: that what has been buried in both the individual and the social psyche creaks to life in the form of "The Other, The Monster" . . .

> . . . that which bourgeois ideology cannot accept but must deal with (as Barthes suggests in *Mythologies*) in one of two ways: either by rejecting it and if possible annihilating it, or by rendering it safe and assimilating it, converting it as far as possible into a replica of itself.

And *what* is repressed is, very largely, sexuality. "The release of sexuality in the horror film is always presented as perverted, monstrous and excessive . . ." — but, moving off *films*, this is precisely how homosexuality and predatory female sexuality are represented in the wider Horror discourse of *newspapers*, *TV* and *people's imaginations*. The monster chained in so many mental dungeons is precisely "unacceptable" sexualities.

This splitting off and projection is, if not exactly a solution, at least one way of dealing with what cannot be contemplated: turning the

Repressed into an Other. But what seems to be particularly threatening about AIDS is that it is linked to the *breakdown* of boundaries. The virus threatens to cross over that border between Other and Self: the threat it poses is not only one of disease but one of dissolution, the contamination of categories. "It" — as a British government poster so anthropomorphically put it — "isn't prejudiced." And, in a kind of analogue to this transgression of social bounds, it also "breaks down" the systems of the body, "letting in" the infections that a functioning immune system keeps firmly out. Thus while on the one hand, enlisted to the codes of narrative order, the virus becomes a coherent subject, with schedules, targets and even an admirable lack of prejudice, on the other it threatens the disintegration of precisely that order of narrative closure which keeps our subjectivity in place — and, in its effects on the body itself, seems to produce the very image of dissolution of the subject, the self as cut out from the world and separate from all that is not-self.

The fear of a dispersal of self-dom can in various ways be linked to the repression of a polymorphous sexuality which — to paraphrase Freud very loosely — is supposedly a necessary component of "adult" heterosexuality. Gay and lesbian sex are not frightening merely because they are perceived as "Other" but precisely because they suggest, or recall, the dissolution of the binary categories on which straight-dom rests. There may be something of this dynamic even *within* gay culture. Returning to the highly symbolic airline steward: "At one time Gaetan had been what every man wanted from gay life; by the time he died, he had become what every man feared." While a narrative may separate the good from the bad, the desired from the feared, the single image or figure can always combine them. Again, categories of meaning break down: and, again, the body provides the appropriate metaphor, as the life-giving substance, blood, "turns against" its "owner". To quote Shilts again: "At any time, without any coherent reason, the virus could emerge from its victims' blood and violently seize their lives." This conjures up an image exactly like the Alien, when it bursts out of someone's stomach: one of the most disturbing moments of the film for, yet again, the bounds of the body are broken.

Julia Kristeva, in *The Powers of Horror*, characterizes the "abject" as something that is neither subject nor object:

There looms, within abjection, one of those violent, dark

revolts of being, directed against a threat that seems to emanate from an exorbitant outside or inside, ejected beyond the scope of the possible, the tolerable, the thinkable. It beseeches, worries and fascinates desire, which, nevertheles, does not let itself be seduced ... What is abject ... is radically excluded and draws me toward the place where meaning collapses ... It is not lack of cleanliness or health that causes abjection but what disturbs identity, system, order. What does not respect borders, positions, rules. The in-between, the ambiguous ...

Unhelpful as I find many of Kristeva's psychoanalytic models, here, drawing heavily on the "dirt as disorder" work of anthropologist Mary Douglas, she describes precisely a dynamic which has a powerful bearing on the Horror scenarios of AIDS. The oscillation between fascination with, and denial of, otherness and difference, the simultaneous wish to know and the wish not to know, all play their part in people's perceptions of AIDS.

How is any of this relevant for people involved with AIDS work? At the ICA conference one speaker asserted that it was a waste of time "looking at advertising and imagery" and that what we should confront was the reality. But the problem is precisely that our experience of reality is always mediated through structures of meaning which, though by no means immutable, actually have a bearing on what we think *is* real, and how we explain and understand it. These in turn have an effect on what we *do* about it. I am particularly concerned to trace the history of some of the genres through which AIDS is perceived because I think it is politically important to realize that AIDS has fitted into a language that was already there, and whose significance is in its structure (origins, goals, etc.) as well as its content. AIDS has not "provoked" all the hysterical responses to it — it has entered an *already* homophobic, blame-oriented culture obsessed with particular types of closed narratives. And no one, gay or straight, left-wing or right-wing, feels that they live in an entirely meaningless universe — although in "reality" we all do. As I have suggested, the body, which is in material terms continuous with that universe, is the point at which structures of meaning become both particularly necessary and particularly easily broken. A study like Susan Sontag's *Illness as*

Metaphor, although about language, has a function very much on the level of the body itself: for in some ways the location and possible deconstruction of those symbolic structures in which the body means, help precisely to give space back to that "reality", whatever it may be, of the body as physical — ridding it, however fleetingly, of what Lacan in a memorable phrase has called the "toxic signifier".

I have tried to suggest some ways of thinking about the perception of AIDS in our culture, precisely because those perceptions stand in the way of confronting a physical reality, and also because they have a bearing on what people do about it and how they *behave*. Terror, whether in a Cronenberg film or a homophobic housing association, and pity, whether in a weepy melodrama or a patronizing tone, are *not* the only emotions available to us (where is ANGER, for example?) but they *are* the ones produced through the centuries-old generic structures that dominate our popular culture, and within it, AIDS speech. I have not used up a lot of space on attacking far-right positions, partly because in the context of this book I didn't think it was necessary, but also because I believe that all of us inhabit mental structures that to a greater or lesser extent need shaking up. AIDS workers are not exempt from this: the Ministering Angel features in some narratives, the All-Knowing Scientist in others — and while these may be infinitely better than Holy Retribution scenarios, it is worth acknowledging that they *are* scenarios, and that what both disturbs them and renders them necessary is the meaninglessness of death.

This takes me back to where I started. But it is not a negative starting point nor, I hope, finishing point. It is only as familiar structures of meaning are shaken and taken apart that new ones can form. And looking at things differently makes it possible to *act* differently. The hackneyed scenarios through which we make sense of many things are challenged by the advent of AIDS. As we find ways to confront the syndrome itself that challenge and the changes it can bring are surely worth rising to.

This essay owes much to two collaborative projects: a course on film genre and the horror film, taught with Barry Curtis at Middlesex Polytechnic, and a season of horror films and melodramas relating to AIDS, entitled *Panic in the Streets*, co-programmed with Mark Finch at the National Film Theatre, London, in August 1988. A dossier from this season comprising an overview plus analyses of each film is available from the Education Department of the British Film Institute.

RICHARD GOLDSTEIN

AIDS AND THE SOCIAL CONTRACT

Every time I heard about another death in the early stages of the epidemic, I would strain to find some basis for a distinction between the deceased and myself: he was a clone, a crisco queen, a midnight sling artist. Then Nathan died of AIDS, and Peter, and Ralph, to whom this piece is dedicated. When it moved in on my friends, the epidemic shattered my presumption of immunity. I, too, was vulnerable, and everything I thought and did about AIDS changed once I faced that fact.

Something like this process is going on in what the American media call the "general public". There is a secret logic Americans apply to people with AIDS: they are sick because they are the Other, and they are the Other because they belong to groups that have always been stigmatized. Every now and then, we read about a woman or child with AIDS, but usually, they are black — another invitation to Otherness for the general public. The disease has brought all sorts of stigma to the surface, and made the fears that any deviance conjures up seem hyper-real. If anything, AIDS has made society less willing to confront those fears, because they suddenly seem so useful as a way to distinguish between people — and acts —that are "risky" or "safe". Rejecting partners who look like they run with junkies or queers is a lot less threatening than mastering the art of condoms. We would rather rely on stigma to protect us than on precautions that would force us to acknowledge that AIDS is not only among us, but of us.

The hot topic in AIDS discussions right now is how efficiently HIV can be transmitted during heterosexual intercourse. The medical answer is by no means clear: about a third of the sex partners of infected IV-drug users in the US have themselves become infected, but nearly all are women. To date, only six men in New York City, which has about half the nation's heterosexual AIDS cases, acquired the virus during straight sex. Whether the ratio will change over time is anybody's guess. The point is that our sense of who is vulnerable to AIDS is based not on conclusive information about the disease, but on assumptions about its victims. Those who believe AIDS could permeate society tend to see carriers as ordinary people who were infected by specific practices. Any act that spreads the disease is potentially dangerous, regardless of its moral meaning. Those who are convinced the risk is low or non-existent tend to see these acts, and the people who perform them, as isolated and perverse. Normal people do not do those things, and therefore, they will be spared. On the fringes of this scenario, AIDS is regarded as a natural process of eliminating the abominable.

Most of us are rationalists in the streets and moralists in the sheets. We look back on the past when people flocked to their churches in times of plague with pity and contempt for those who thought piety would spare them. Yet we act as if only corrupt acts, performed by corrupt people can transmit HIV. What's more, we proceed as if the corrupt and virtuous never meet in bed. In this incantation of immunity, I hear echoes of my own denial. Every gay man alive is Ishmael, with a tale to tell about the infinite capacity of human beings to deny what they cannot feel or see. But the stigma that surrounds homosexuality makes it hard for heterosexuals to act as if my witness applies to them. Few of my straight friends are compelled to ponder the question that has haunted me ever since I saw it plastered on a wall in Greenwich Village: "Why him and not me?"

This is a timeless question. In the West, we try to answer it by referring to an unwritten charter with a checkered history: the social contract. Its terms are often glibly applied to the inequities of race and class, but when it comes to illness —especially infectious illness — the social contract has been used as a cudgel against the infirm. Yet, it is the standard by which public health policy is measured, and its terms are embedded in the rhetoric of countless AIDS commissions, which seek to "balance public safety and personal liberty". In America, these are buzz-words for an AIDS policy that reconciles the demands of the infected with the fears of the worried well. The assumption is that both groups are equally needy of protection. They are not. The power differential between people with AIDS and people afraid of AIDS is the most salient fact about this epidemic. That disparity is sustained by stigma, and we will never be able to craft a just response to AIDS until we confront the role stigma plays in defining this disease and creating a doomed, dangerous victim class.

Stigma, the Plague and AIDS

Susan Sontag has observed that illness is made infinitely harder to bear by its affinity for metaphor. We pity the afflicted and simultaneously shun them, regardless of the actual danger they pose. In times of plague, the entire range of stigma is called into play in the service of public safety, and one is reminded that the word itself first entered our vocabulary as a description of the marks and signs of illness. For medieval Christians, lepers and victims of bubonic plague were literally stigmatized. This diagnosis persists in the contemporary notion that many illnesses — from cancer to ulcers — are expressions of a character flaw.

If the sick are often stigmatized, they are also, in many cases, dispensable. In the best of times, the temptation to ignore the vital interests of some patients is why we have an elaborate code of medical consent. But when plague strikes, we discover that there are no rights so inalienable that they cannot be subordinated to the greater good. Isolating the infected began with leprosy in the Middle Ages. Once the concept of latent infection gained acceptance, the quarantine expanded to include anyone who might have been exposed to infectious diseases. The pages of Defoe are filled with the howls of those locked up in their homes — healthy people trapped with dying relatives or spouses. Finally, entire cities are stigmatized. Murder is not uncommon, as refugees wander the countryside in search of food and shelter. In the plague zone, all the amenities of death —the rituals of nursing, praying, and memorializing — are sacrificed to the imperatives of corpse disposal. Merrymaking is banned, and the stench of gunpowder and vinegar hangs in the air.

So far, our response to AIDS has been governed by the distinctly modern assumption that epidemics can be contained. The periodic demands to crack down on commercial sex notwithstanding, very little has changed about the quality of public life in New York. Every now and then, there is a bizarre reminder that the city is suffering a collective trauma; as when medical waste, some of it contaminated with HIV, washed up on local beaches last summer, forcing them to close. But by and large, the anguish of the afflicted and loathing of the well are artfully privatized. Visitors would hardly know that New York City is in the grip of a health emergency. Partly, this reflects the fact that AIDS is a plague in slow motion; we are witnessing a protracted period of latency with no real idea of how far the infection will extend. But our obliviousness also derives from the conviction that AIDS is a disease of the deviant. This image persists because, in America, the virus did initially appear to single out groups — and acts — regarded as contaminating. Many illnesses transform their victims into a stigmatized class, but AIDS is the first epidemic to take stigmatized classes and make them victims. Not even syphilis was so precise.

Worse still, AIDS is demonstrably infectious. So carriers are marked both by their Otherness and by the common humanity they are denied. They can infect anyone, though they themselves are infected because they are not just anyone. This paradox amplifies the fear and denial that always surround disease. AIDS is not just contagious; it is polluting. To catch this disease is to have your identity stolen; to be lowered, body and soul, into the pit of deviance. This is true even for an "innocent victim", since, once stigma attaches to an illness, it ceases to be about behaviour. Anyone with AIDS becomes the Other. And since anyone can be made Other by this disease, deviance itself must be contagious. The most cherished components of personal identity can, irrationally and abruptly, be revoked. This may explain why, though a majority of Americans say they oppose discrimination against people with AIDS, 26 per cent of those polled by Gallup last month still fear drinking from a glass or eating food prepared by an infected person. What people fear from casual contact is not so much the disease as its very real power to pollute.

Stigma is the reason an AIDS patient in North Carolina, being transferred from one hospital to another, arrived wrapped in a body bag with a small air tube to allow breathing. Stigma is the reason a plane carrying demonstrators to the gay rights march on Washington in October 1987 was fumigated after landing. Stigma is the reason a social worker in the Bronx must regularly visit a healthy child whose parents have succumbed to AIDS, because no neighbour will comb her hair. Polls tell us people are more "enlightened" about AIDS. What people are becoming enlightened about is transmission modes, but the impact of stigma remains poorly understood. It is rarely mentioned in discussions of AIDS prevention, though the fear of being stigmatized is often the reason infected people have sex without revealing the danger to their partners. It is seldom raised in discussions of testing, though stigma plays a part in determining who will be screened — and why people resist screening in the first place. Stigma has always been a factor in mass detentions; the incarceration of Japanese-Americans during World War II had everything to do with their Otherness. Yet, opponents of proposals to isolate AIDS carriers often argue their case on the less contentious grounds of cost efficiency. To acknowledge that so much of what we fear stems from the conviction that AIDS is a disease of people with "spoiled identities" (Erving Goffman's phrase) would threaten the validity of these categories. So liberals try to separate AIDS the infection from AIDS the stigma, as if, by skirting the issue, they can transcend it. But in fact an unexamined stigma is free to expand. Because it is not an objective condition, but a relationship between the normal and the deviant, stigma ripples out from the reviled to include their neighbourhoods, even the cities where they congregate. In the USA, whole postal districts have been marked by some insurance companies as AIDS zones, and when rumours about a famous fashion designer circulated, the concern was whether people would still be seen in clothing that bears his name. The stigma of AIDS has the capacity to reinvigorate ancient stereotypes, not just about sexuality but about race and urbanity. And no city in America is more vulnerable to this conjunction of biases than New York. Half its AIDS cases are among IV-drug users, most of them heterosexual and non-white. Unless a treatment is found the death toll in black and Hispanic neighbourhoods will eventually approach what it is today in Kinshasa. As the boundaries of infection extend, more and more of us will live in fear of being stigmatized. And in the end, it will not matter who is actually vulnerable. The entire city will bear the brand of AIDS.

And its cost. By 1991, the New York State Department of Health estimates, 10 per cent of hospital beds in the city will be occupied by AIDS patients. Some administrators think that figure will be more like one in four — a prospect that terrifies them, since the city's hospitals are already operating at 90 per cent capacity. Moreover, because so many AIDS patients in New York are IV-users, they stay in hospital longer than AIDS patients in other cities, and their infections are more expensive to treat. These patients are already putting an enormous strain on scarce medical resources. As the gap between supply and demand becomes acute, a kind of sifting process could well emerge, along with violations of privacy, autonomy, and informed consent — fragile concepts of medical ethics that were not formally codified until the Nuremberg trials after World War II. The mounting despair of physicians in the face of demands that cannot be met from patients who cannot be saved is bound to affect the practice of medicine for all New Yorkers. The burnout is already leading to an exodus of doctors — as has often happened in cities besieged by plague. But New York is only the focal point of an epidemic that will soon make its presence felt in every American city. A recent study sponsored by the Centers for Disease Control predicts that, by 1991, the bill for AIDS will be $8.5 billion in medical costs alone — more money than is spent on any group of patients except for victims of automobile accidents. By 1991, the "indirect costs", in terms of productivity, of a disease that kills people in their prime will be more than $55 billion — 12 per cent of the indirect cost of all illnesses. AIDS will be among the top ten killers of Americans, and the leading killer of people between the ages of twenty-five to forty-four. "People do not seem to realize that, beyond compassion, there's a real self-interest in controlling AIDS, because we do not have the resources to handle this and all the other diseases," says medical ethicist Carol Levine, executive director of the Citizens Commission on AIDS, a private non-profit group. "Everyone who gets sick will pay the price for thinking people can be separated."

Most of us still think AIDS is happening to someone else. It's not. AIDS is happening to some of *us*, and in some places, many of us. In the Bronx today, 6 per cent of all women over twenty-five using a pre-natal clinic, and 14 per cent of all patients who had blood drawn in an emergency room, test positive for antibodies. One in sixty-one babies born in public hospitals in New York City is carrying HIV. Are they junkies? Are they faggots? Are they niggers? Are they us?

Response to the Risk

Where epidemics are concerned, the race, class, and sexuality of carriers has always played a major part in how they are cared for and how dangerous they seem. Isolation, incarceration, the destruction of whole neighbourhoods — all these public health measures have been practised at one time or another in the USA, almost exclusively against poor, non-white, or sexually "disreputable" people. AIDS hysteria is a throwback to a politics of public health we thought we'd put behind us — the "purity crusade" that flourished in America during the early part of this century, constructing the reality of prohibition and the ideal of abstinence. It turns out that the hygiene police have been lying in wait for a crisis: AIDS is their opportunity.

This most social of diseases has occasioned the most political of responses. One has only to ponder the thundering silence in the US Senate whenever Jesse Helms rises to rail about "safe sodomy". Every plan for prevention, every push for treatment and research funds, is guided by ideological assumptions. The image of a person with AIDS determines who we think is guilty or innocent, where we fix blame for the epidemic, and whether we support a policy of education and volition or one of regulation and repression. Where we place ourselves in relation to the stigma surrounding this disease determines what we think is necessary to protect ourselves: whether we think laws are needed to identify, and if necessary, isolate HIV carriers; whether "innocent" people ought to take risks on their behalf. It is not the extent of risk but its source that made a judge in California recently rule that a teacher of deaf children could be removed from the classroom because he carries HIV antibodies. It's the image of the carrier that makes physicians and police insist on taking extraordinary precautions. In both these cases, people who might ordinarily place themselves in considerable peril shrink from the relatively minor danger posed by those who carry the HIV virus. In some American cities, police who risk their lives in pursuit of criminals wear rubber gloves during gay rights demonstrations. At some US hospitals, surgeons who run a high risk of contracting hepatitis (a blood-borne virus that infects twenty-five thousand health workers — and kills three hundred — every year) refuse to operate on people with HIV. There's not a single reported case of HIV being transmitted in the operating room; only doctors and nurses who care for AIDS patients day after day, and lab technicians who are constantly exposed to the live virus, have been infected in the line of duty. Nevertheless, Dr Ronald M. Abel, who has emerged as a spokesman for surgeons refusing to operate on people with HIV, justifies such decisions on the spurious grounds that they commit not only the physicians but "dozens of operating-room assistants to a high degree of risk." Though no policeman has ever been infected by a suspect, Phil Caruso, president of the Patrolmen's Benevolent Association, a labour union in New York City, urges his members to: "do whatever is necessary to protect your life and health in any police situation, be it a shoot-out or the handling of an AIDS sufferer, each of which is a potentially lethal proposition."

Carol Levine calls this refusal to deal with the relatively manageable hazards of AIDS "a disjunction of risk". She maintains that "what people are afraid of is not dying, but what happens before." A cop who is killed rescuing a baby from the ruins of a collapsed building becomes a hero. A doctor who risks his life to treat a victim of radiation poisoning, as happened recently in Brazil, makes the news. But HIV invests all its hosts with stigma. Doctors carrying HIV have lost their practices; a policeman with AIDS could well imagine his peers abandoning him — and his family. Parents told that a classmate with AIDS poses no threat to their children might reason that, even if the children's safety is not at stake, their normalcy is. Shunned by other children, they may become bearers of another stigma. And for what? "When you voluntarily assume a risk, it fits your self-image," says Levine. "But this is a risk you did not bargain for — and it's being brought to you by people you're not crazy about — so it's perceived as unacceptable." Though AIDS has been dehomosexualized in the popular imagination, its origins as a "gay plague" continue to haunt the affected — and prevent us from acknowledging that, on a global scale, most people with AIDS are heterosexuals and their children. "What's the hardest thing about getting AIDS?" goes the joke among gay men. "Convincing your mother that you're Haitian." This is a nasty gag about the hierarchy of stigma, and few Haitians would be amused. Each stigma feels like the ultimate injustice, and each oppression seems unique. But the odium attached to race and sexuality actually reflects a single process, whose function is to organize and validate the norm. Anyone can fall prey to such a beast —the "innocent victim" along with the defiled. The irony about health workers demanding that their patients be tested for HIV antibodies is that it will surely lead to a demand by their patients that doctors and nurses take the test — with inevitable penalties for those infected.

Taking the Test

I was surprised by the anxiety testing provokes in heterosexuals, until I realized that nearly everyone I know has had a relationship with someone who might be infected. In any urban population, most people who take the test pass through a psychic rite that has less to do with fear of death than with the consequences of a positive result: guilt over the past, rage at the present, fear of the future. That fear must include not only the disease but disclosure — and the range of rejections that might ensue. Yet it is seldom remarked that, for anyone in a vulnerable group, taking the test is an act of enormous courage. The only controversy is over whether such people should be forced to know their antibody status — and in this debate, the anguish of an AIDS "suspect" is easily subordinated to that great equalizer, the common good. Stigma determines whose interests are expendable. "You always assume the test will happen to someone else," says Levine. "Left to their own devices, most people do not want to know."

That may be wise. As the *New York Times* acknowledged, the potential for inaccuracy in the general population is high enough to make mass testing a "treacherous paradox". Yet certain populations are expected to bear the uncertainty: soldiers, aliens applying for amnesty, Job Corps workers, and in some hospitals where state law permits, candidates for surgery. Recently, the Senate voted to require all veterans in hospitals to "mandatorily offer antibody testing" — an interesting euphemism, since patients who refuse the offer would risk being treated like a person with AIDS. (Turning down the test is, in itself, a stigmatizing experience, because it implies that you have had reason to suspect ... you may have had sex with ... or might even be ...!) What these groups have in common is not the danger they might pose to others, but the fact that they depend on public institutions. In America everyone who relies on the government must expect to forfeit some basic rights. There is talk of subjecting other populations, such as welfare recipients, stigmatized by their dependence to mandatory testing. An old adage must be dusted off in the current crisis: "If you prick us, do we not bleed?"

Commonality in Stigma

It takes a leap of consciousness to see the connection between one stigma and another. Gay men and IV-users face each other across a vast behavioural divide. But both cultures are based on behaviour — indeed, on an act of penetration deemed illicit. Both deviate from the norms of ecstasy, and invest their deviance with enormous significance, using it to foster intimate bonds and a "lifestyle" with its own slang and gait. Both exist as distinct groups within every class, though the drug culture flourishes in the ghetto, as a symbol of its vulnerability, and gay culture is most militant in bourgeois society. Of course, shooting heroin has profound implications for one's health and security, while homosexuality, per se, does not. And the drug culture is a violent, haunted environment. But it *is* a culture, and though we need to keep its damage in mind, we also must wonder how much the antisocial behaviour associated with IV use stems from stigma and from the stranglehold of dealers. Freed from both these sources of oppression, the IV-user might re-emerge as a citizen, and we might have to reconsider what the word "junkie" really means.

"It seems that some real change in the cultural norms is going to be necessary," says Don Des Jarlais, a behavioural researcher at the New York State Division of Substance Abuse Services. "Society will have to make a decision that the chance of spreading this virus is so great, and drug users play so crucial a part in that spread, that we cannot simply allow them to die of AIDS or make a rule that they must stop using drugs in order *not* to die of AIDS."

Rescuing the IV-user may involve some of the same techniques that have worked in the gay community. Perhaps the sharing of needles can be understood in the same context as anal sex — as an ecstatic act that enhances social solidarity. "Within the subculture, the running partner becomes the substitute for family," Des Jarlais writes. "It would be considered a major insult to refuse to use one's partner's works . . . [or] share one's own works . . . . It would undermine the teamwork and synchronicity of intense experience that are the bases of the running-buddy relationship." One answer is to provide the IV-equivalent of a condom: bleach kits or clean needles. Contrary to the assumption that drug users are oblivious to AIDS, Des Jarlais reports that the epidemic is "a topic of 'grave' concern among IV-drug users" in several cities, and that they "want to learn how to protect themselves against exposure." Safe injection is as central to the humanistic AIDS agenda as safe sex.

Des Jarlais has observed more ambivalence among drug users than among gay men about discussing AIDS prevention with their sexual partners. It may be fear of abandonment that stands in the way of candour. "Most IV-users have their primary relationship with a non-drug-using partner," says Des Jarlais. The dependence for food, shelter, and money — not to mention emotional security — can be intense. "When you have a pair like that, there's no symmetricality of risk. To bring up the subject of AIDS points to the disparity in the relationship. Half the time, the partner using condoms gets abandoned by his female lover. So it's easier to practise safe sex with a casual partner than in a long-term relationship." Surveys have found the same phenomenon among gay men, but the likelihood that either partner could be carrying the virus makes mutual safety part of their bond.

Most gay men have other advantages — not just race and class, but organization. One has only to imagine what the American response to AIDS would be like if the gay rights movement did not exist. There is no annual pride parade of drug users, no press that circulates among them, and their advocacy organizations, at least in New York, are severely underfunded. Organizing IV-users may enable their culture to preserve its members by altering the rituals of risk, much as gay men have altered theirs. It may empower users to strike back at oppressive dealers and lobby for access to meaningful treatment. But funding this liberation means overcoming what Des Jarlais calls "an empathy barrier".

So far, the support system for people with AIDS has done more to break down this barrier than any church or public agency. About a quarter of the clients at Gay Men's Health Crisis are non-gay, and many groups for "body positives" (as carriers now call themselves) are integrated. But most gay men and IV-users still cannot imagine that each other's identities might spring from a shared perspective. As Erving Goffman writes: "Persons with different stigmas are [affected] in an appreciably similar way." AIDS forces us to confront this commonality. The "innocent" black woman infected by her lover, the gay man whose class has always insulated him, the addict abandoned in a hospital ward — all were victims of stigma before they became victims of disease. And though they may live (and die) in utter contempt for each other's deviations from the norm, they are implicated in each other's fate. What happens to the prostitute can happen to the amateur; what they do to the junkie they can do to the fag.

In hospital, everyone looks like the Other. An AIDS ward in New

York City is no different, except that, in a public hospital, it might be filled with black people. I walked through one such ward on assignment, trying not to look too hard at the flesh bundles in the beds. Finally, I took a long peek at a black woman in her late thirties, propped up on pillows, surrounded by tissues and magazines. She had the gaunt intensity that people in the late stages of AIDS often get, as if her entire being were confined to the eyes. I stopped seeing her race and sex, both of which are, in some sense, alien to me. Instead, I saw my lover. She resembled him, not as he was, but as he might be if he ever got AIDS. I walked on quickly, struggling to fight the welling up of tears.

That night, I dreamt I was leaving my apartment for work. There was a corpse outside the door.

The Social Contract

"Love," writes Martin Buber, "is the responsibility of an I for a thou." In social terms, this suggests that the bond between citizens is as essential to human development as the bond between lovers, or between parent and child. The social contract is a codification of that bond — an agreement to form a government that sustains us. There is a simultaneous obligation to protect each other, discharged through duties and limits on behaviour which we accept as a fair price for the welfare of the community. Without this compact no individual can survive.

When a health crisis strikes, Buber's equation becomes demonstrable: the mutual obligation of the infected and the uninfected is the responsibility of an I for a thou. As we confront the limits of freedom, the ego becomes collectivized, and the community, an abstraction in ordinary times, becomes the tangible sum of its parts. An ethic of inclusiveness makes personal sacrifice not only bearable, but unremarkable. One simply does what is necessary, because, as Camus writes, "the only means of fighting a plague is common decency."

The gay community has gone through just such a process in the face of AIDS. It has reshaped itself to care for its own, and rejected behaviour once regarded as the mark of liberation. But gay people have every reason to mistrust the social contract. It has always been enforced at their expense. For homosexuals, "public health" has been a rationale for stigma. They are among the usual suspects rounded up in panics over sexually transmitted diseases. AIDS threatens to revive this tradition of hygiene-programmes on a much more devastating scale. William Buckley, a prominent rightwing TV commentator, recently suggested that people with AIDS be tattooed on the forearm and buttocks to warn the uninfected. This shows how easily the technocratic imagination can conjure up what Goffman calls a "stigma symbol". Every now and then someone hatches a gothic variation on Buckley's scheme; the urge literally to stigmatize the infected will not die. A new book, *Aids in America: Our Chances, Our Choices*, recommends "discreet genital tattooing" — just outside the urethra for men, just inside the labia minora for women. Such proposals are always couched in the rhetoric of reason and equity, as if they would apply to anyone who happened to be infected. But in reality, they can only be enacted on people whose freedom is already precarious. IV-users and prostitutes are eminently detainable, and the parole granted homosexuals can easily be revoked.

It's a mark of my generation to regard the social contract as fraught with bad faith. But AIDS cannot be stopped without a compact among citizens, which is enforced by the government. It demands that we renegotiate the terms, infusing the contract with an expanded sense of equity — and empathy. "Our best weapon against AIDS," writes Dan Beauchamp in his book *The Health of the Republic*, "would be a public health policy resting on the right to be different in fundamental choices and the democratic community as 'one body' in matters of the common health. This new policy would mean the right of every individual to fundamental autonomy, as in abortion and sexual orientation, while viewing health and safety as a common good whose protection (through restrictions on liberty) promotes community and the common health."

Under a new social contract, we could talk about the limits on personal freedom in a time of plague; the need for vulnerable people to know their antibody status or act as if they are seropositive; the duty to protect your partners and inform others at risk. But saving lives also means setting limits on moralism: confronting the full range of human sexuality, including its expression in the erotics of shooting up; promoting the use of any implement — condoms, needles — that slows the spread of AIDS (if anything, we will have to demand better implements); breaking down barriers of sexism that dispose women to infection and men to secrecy. AIDS renders both the liberationist mentality and the moralistic world view obsolete. But so far, only the sexual revolution has been criticized — and in highly moralistic terms. The public health profession has beaten back the most savage proposals for dealing with AIDS, but it is neither powerful enough, nor militant enough, to stand up to political and social conservatism. Ethicists fill monographs with their vision of the social contract, while the usual bad bargain is forged by church and state. And the epidemic goes on, as sexually transmitted diseases always have, stoked by shame and secrecy. But in the age of AIDS, social justice cannot be promoted in purely pragmatic terms. It is too easy to imagine the majority protected by the erotic segregation that pervades American society. The danger is not that AIDS will wipe our species off the planet, but that it will wipe out people most of us already hate — and that is a moral as well as a medical crisis. "My worst fear," says Beauchamp, "is not the concentration camps but a kind of paralysis, in which people will just be left to cope." As a professor of public health in North Carolina, Beauchamp sees the epidemic not as an incarnation of the holocaust (with which it is often wrongly compared), but as a "new civil war". The danger for him lies in "splitting off another chunk of the Republic", condemning hundreds of thousands of Americans, and on a global scale millions, to expendability. The wages of this sin is not only death, but "a kind of amnesia about who we are and who we want to be."

Every society is haunted by events that expose the gap between who we are and who we want to be. They may happen to other people, but they reveal us to ourselves. Hiroshima and Vietnam are watersheds in American culture because they were moral as well as military conflagrations. These two events shaped my generation. I believe AIDS will define the next.

TOM STODDARD

PARADOX AND PARALYSIS

An Overview of the American Response to AIDS

Acquired Immune Deficiency Syndrome (AIDS) challenges more than medicine. Because it is deadly, because it continues to spread quickly, because it is linked to the controversial subjects of sex and drugs, and also because, in the developed world at least, it arose first among gay men and heroin addicts, it provokes deep and complicated feelings in nearly everyone, and those feelings when extended across a society, have political and social consequences. As AIDS moves across the world, it tests each country's ability to act responsibly — or even sanely — in the face of catastrophe.

This short article will attempt to outline the way in which the United States of America has responded, or failed to respond, to the unique challenges of this modern epidemic. The article will look particularly at the way in which government and the private or voluntary sector in the United States have divided up the tasks imposed by the emergence of AIDS, and then proceeded to perform those tasks, with the hope that the US example will be instructive to other countries that have not yet had to face the brunt of the epidemic.

An analysis of this kind is particularly difficult with a nation as large, and as culturally and politically diverse, as the United States. This article will not attempt to relate the history of AIDS in the United States, even in summary form, but will instead identify patterns and themes in the country's overall response to the crisis since AIDS was first recognized in 1981.

The following four paradoxes will help to give the flavour of the American response to date for those readers who live outside the United States:

1. News about AIDS is everywhere in the United States. Newspapers, periodicals, television and radio stations all report regularly on AIDS, dedicating far more attention to this subject than to any other health problem. Nonetheless, many Americans are still ignorant of such elementary facts about AIDS as the ways in which the Human Immunodeficiency Virus (HIV), which is believed to cause AIDS, is transmitted from one person to another. In a Gallup poll released in March 1988, nearly 40 per cent of American workers accepted the proposition (which is totally without scientific basis) that they might catch the virus through food served in the company cafeteria. The ignorance of the public is, to some extent, driven by fear, as in Arcadia, Florida, where unknown malefactors set fire to the home of three haemophiliac boys with HIV in their blood. The boys posed no threat to any of their playmates, but the neighbours seem to have been so fearful for their children that they simply could not accept the reassurances of the experts. The persistence of such irrational fears is co-extensive with the amount of media attention.

2. Most political leaders in the United States have voiced their commitment to overcoming AIDS. President Reagan himself characterized AIDS as the nation's foremost health problem. Yet, seven years after the identification of the illness and four years after the discovery of HIV, there is still no national plan on AIDS. The primary burden of the illness has fallen, institutionally, on the fifty state governments and the localities within them, particularly those on the east and west coasts, most of which lack the resources to address the issue adequately. President Reagan did, in 1987, create a special presidential commission on AIDS, or, as he put it, "the Human Immunodeficiency Virus Epidemic," but after the commission issued its final report in June 1988, he simply ignored its principal recommendations.

3. In the absence of decisive action by the government, particularly at the federal level, hundreds of private organizations have sprung into being to provide services to people with AIDS, and to others touched by AIDS. The prototype is Gay Men's Health Crisis in New York City, which began in someone's living room in 1981 and now, a mere seven years later, has an annual budget of more than $10 million and a staff of more than one hundred people. Although miraculous in their creation and heroic in their achievements, these

organizations are limited in what they can do and are generally ill-equipped to address the future trends in the epidemiology of AIDS. AIDS is likely to become less a disease of the white gay men who were the first publicized persons to develop the illness, and more a disease of intravenous drug users, most of whom are poor and black or Hispanic. In New York City, for example, drug users and their sexual partners now account for a majority of the newly diagnosed cases. The name "Gay Men's Health Crisis" in itself suggests the difficulty that organization will have in shifting its focus, assuming it should choose to do so. (New York City is also home to an organization called the Minority Task Force on AIDS, but the group has one-tenth of the budget and one-tenth of the number of employees of Gay Men's Health Crisis; it also receives considerably less attention from the press and from government.)

4. It is illegal for most private employers in the United States to fire, demote, or harass people with AIDS and people with HIV infection, unless an employee simply cannot do the job. Most states, as well as the federal government, have statutes forbidding discrimination on account of a worker's "handicap" or "disability", and increasingly these statutes have been interpreted to extend to AIDS. Consequently, while some employers faced with the issue of AIDS have acted stupidly or maliciously, and discrimination does without question exist, it is less than systematic — with one notorious exception. The federal government itself does discriminate against people with AIDS and HIV infection. The government now tests for HIV antibodies all applicants for military service, for the Peace Corps (which sends volunteers abroad to teach skills), and for residential placements in the Job Corps (which trains poor teenagers for employment), and rejects those with positive results. The government also requires tests of all Foreign Service officers and their spouses, all immigrants, and all prisoners subject to its jurisdiction. Thus, the federal government views itself as exempt from the rules imposed on other American employers.

As these four paradoxes imply, America has responded to AIDS with confusion and inconsistency. The picture so far is an extraordinary jumble of images, with signs of great courage and hope — the growth of Gay Men's Health Crisis, for example — beside symbols of failure — most prominently, President Reagan's virtual abdication of responsibility on the issue. The achievements have come largely from outside the government, as private individuals and organizations have discovered the problem and sought to address it. Within the government, especially in Washington, the response has been clumsy, feeble and tardy. Official Washington has by now at least acknowledged publicly that AIDS is an epidemic, and one full of peril, but it is still unable to put together a strategy to overcome it. A nation that devised Project Apollo, the Marshall Plan, and the Manhattan Project has been unable to agree with itself on what to do about any aspect of the crisis posed by the Human Immunodeficiency Virus. The government cannot even achieve a consensus on what to tell ordinary citizens about the virus, with some officials urging warnings that are explicit and others advocating more circumspect messages for reasons of propriety, personal morality, or politics.

This failure of leadership is critical because of the enormity of the crisis in the United States. The United States is the epicentre of AIDS in the developed world. Apart from Africa, which has an epidemiology of its own, the United States was the first place in the world with a substantial AIDS caseload. And with currently more than seventy thousand identified cases, it still accounts for two-thirds of the world's caseload outside Africa. The statistical future is even grimmer than the past. The federal government believes that at least one and a half million Americans have HIV in their blood. Unless science can find a treatment more effective than those now available, most of these people will die premature, HIV-related deaths.

I should add that the American system of government does not lend itself to the efficient — or speedy — resolution of problems. The American federal structure favours stability over change, and diversity over uniformity. Basic services, including public education and public health, rest primarily in the hands of the states and localities, not the federal government. Even at the federal level power is dispersed. The president can propose legislation to Congress, but can rarely force his will on that body, particularly when, as now, it is controlled by the opposition. And the courts hold a potential constitutional checkmate over the actions of both the president and Congress that is unique to the West. Furthermore, the private sector plays a much larger role in American life than in any other developed country. Services that elsewhere belong to the public sector, such as gas, electricity, air travel, broadcasting, and telephones, are provided in the United States by private companies, often in competition with one another. Health care falls in this category. Most Americans obtain health care through private contracts with insurance companies and "health maintenance organizations". The government covers only the elderly and the very poor, and even for them not all forms of care. Under such a system, change comes about only with difficulty, even in the face of an emergency.

Any comprehensive national strategy on AIDS would necessarily centre on four goals: the discovery of a cure; adequate care for the afflicted; the prevention of further spread of HIV; and the elimination of unfair discrimination against those connected with the virus. Sadly, in every one of these areas, the American response to date has been short-sighted and inadequate.

The Search for a Cure

Even in decentralized and highly privatized America, the task of finding a cure must be the responsibility of the federal government. The federal Department of Health and Human Services shelters several agencies designed to promote the development of new drugs and treatments, especially the Food and Drug Administration (FDA) and the National Institutes of Health (NIH). These agencies often work with private companies and universities in their investigations. Under ordinary circumstances, the system of drug development and approval works very slowly. Federal approval for sale of a new drug takes, on average, eight years from the beginning of the first test. Until that time, the drug is generally unavailable to the public, even for a patient facing death whose doctor is prepared to use the drug.

Until recently these agencies had shown slight interest in AIDS, and very little concern over the slowness of the investigative process or the unavailability of a drug until the government gives final approval for its use. In 1986, some reporters and politicians raised questions about the federal government's approach to drug development in light of promising rumours about an anti-viral compound known as azdothymidine (AZT). Their inquiries, together with increasingly encouraging reports from the investigators, moved the FDA and NIH to accelerate rapidly the entire procedure for that particular drug, and AZT was eventually licensed for sale to some, but not all people with AIDS, in the spring of 1987. (It is now available on a wider basis, although its extremely high cost still makes it unavailable to some HIV-infected individuals who wish to use the drug.)

AZT may help to retard replication of the virus, but it is not a cure, and is toxic to some patients. Since its approval, private organizations serving people with AIDS have voiced ever louder — and ever angrier — dissatisfaction with the way in which federal agencies have approached other possible treatments. Indeed, a number of private organizations, such as Project Inform in San Francisco, now advise people with AIDS or HIV on substances not approved by the FDA, and some have surreptitiously helped them to get the drugs from other countries, or from illicit domestic sources. Frustration over federal indifference has also prompted the creation of private organizations that initiate or assist in the testing of treatments outside the typical research channels, such as the Community Research Initiative in New York. Private impatience has in addition greatly spurred charitable donations to a private organization called the American Foundation for AIDS Research (AmFAR), which awards grants of its own to scientists investigating possible treatments for AIDS. In the fiscal year 1985, AmFAR gave research grants totalling, $1,512,278. In the fiscal year 1988 — a mere three years later — it will give $7,200,000.

After several years of criticism and defiance, the FDA in particular has at last begun to bend. In July 1988, the agency's commissioner announced that people with AIDS would be permitted to import for their personal use small quantities of substances only available abroad. The next month he agreed to relax restrictions on an experimental drug for pneumocystis carinii pneumonia, the opportunistic infection that results in the most deaths from AIDS.

But these developments have come much later than they should have, or would have, had the White House taken an interest in the matter. Moreover, they cannot outweigh the persistent refusal of the federal government to adequately fund research into AIDS. Both the Institute of Medicine of the National Academy of Sciences, which is an independent organization funded in part by the federal government, and the president's own commission on AIDS have called for substantial additional federal funding of the national research and development agencies.

Whether these recommendations will be followed may become

clearer in the course of 1989, but there is reason to fear yet more inaction. In the meantime, AMFAR, the Community Research Initiative, Project Inform and other private groups have sought to fill the gaps in federal activity. They, rather than any federal agencies, have pointed the way for those in search of a cure.

Care for the Sick and Infected

Almost alone in the developed world (South Africa is the other exception), the United States offers no comprehensive national health service to its citizens. Health care in the US is a patchwork of programmes, some private and some public, that serve some Americans reasonably well and some very badly or not at all. Most Americans assure health care for themselves and their families through participation in group health insurance plans offered by their employers. Those who are unemployed or self-employed, and those whose employers do not offer them a health plan, must provide for themselves or rely on whatever services, if any, are offered by their local governments.

AIDS has not altered this basic fact of American life. But it has brought attention to the current inequities, and helped build support for public health insurance. (In the summer of 1988, Massachusetts became the first state to guarantee health insurance for all residents.) The changing epidemiology of AIDS will assist that process. AIDS, especially in the north-eastern states, is increasingly an illness afflicting intravenous drug users and therefore the poor —those who, because they have no private insurance, must turn to the government. In a city like New York, with nearly a quarter of the country's AIDS cases and perhaps four hundred thousand people infected with HIV, the costs are soaring. Federal intervention may be the only possible solution short of abandonment of the city and its caseload.

While hundreds of private, local organizations have arisen across the country in the past seven years, to meet the needs of people with AIDS and people at special risk from AIDS, these organizations, with very few exceptions, do not and cannot provide medical care directly. Gay Men's Health Crisis in New York City was the first to do so and is still the model. The organization informs and counsels about AIDS, HIV infection, and their consequences. It links people in need with volunteer companions. It offers recreation and legal assistance. It produces brochures and films. It lobbies in the city council, in the state legislature, and to a more limited extent in Congress. It does not, however, run medical facilities or residences for people with AIDS, and would quickly sink under the work-load if it attempted to. Furthermore, as its name indicates, it arose from and still addresses primarily the concerns of gay men. Because of its history, focus, and name, it is not well-suited to meeting the needs of other people with AIDS or HIV infection.

The Prevention of Further Spread

In June 1988, the United States Government mailed to every American household a pamphlet about AIDS. The language was generally straightforward, but at times euphemistic and equivocal; the pamphlet warned, for example, of "sex with someone you don't know well" without distinguishing between sexual acts involving penetration, which may be dangerous, and sexual conduct without penetration (so-called "safer sex"), which generally is not.

This pamphlet constitutes the principal effort by the federal government to inform the American people about AIDS. It has not been the sole attempt. The federal Centers for Disease Control have given money to private organizations to teach about AIDS, and the surgeon general has talked repeatedly and frankly to the press about AIDS. But the federal government's role has been largely incidental to the work of the private sector. Privately-owned entities have taught the American people about AIDS: not-for-profit corporations like Gay Men's Health Crisis, small film companies like AIDSfilms, and the country's tangle of news outlets.

The disparate, decentralized nature of AIDS education in the United States has had its advantages. The USA is so massive and complex a country that AIDS affects different sectors of the population in different ways; the concerns, needs, and perspectives of gay men differ substantially from those of intravenous drug users. For instance, the sociology of gay men who live in Salt Lake City does not conform to the patterns of the gay male subculture in New York City. But all the individual efforts taken together cannot substitute for a vigorous and cohesive national campaign to communicate certain basic themes to the country as a whole. And any national campaign on AIDS ought to convey more than medical facts and advice. It should, for instance, counsel against unfair treatment or stigmatization of people with HIV. By this broader standard, the federal government has failed totally. Apart from the surgeon general's avuncular admonitions, federal officials have been largely silent. President Reagan himself has been almost entirely absent from the national discussions about AIDS.

A full effort to arrest spread of the virus would embrace, in addition to the dissemination of information, counselling and voluntary testing programmes for people who fear they may be infected, and a campaign against the use of intravenous drugs. Projects of both kinds do exist in the United States, but without substantial federal support. A bill to fund HIV testing centres has yet to pass the Congress. And although the government does furnish some money for drug treatment facilities, the inadequacy of its appropriations is appalling. In the state of New Jersey, for instance, where most AIDS cases arise from the use of drugs, the present drug treatment programmes can accommodate only four thousand of an estimated forty thousand drug users.

The Elimination of Discrimination
The President's Commission on the Human Immunodeficiency Virus Epidemic called in its final report for a broad federal statute to outlaw discrimination against people with AIDS and HIV infection, and also for a presidential order forbidding discrimination within the federal government. James D. Watkins, who headed the commission, was adamant on this issue. In a press conference in June 1988 he characterized discrimination as "the most significant obstacle to progress in controlling the AIDS epidemic," arguing that so long as discrimination persisted, it would deter people from seeking testing, counselling, and care. The President however, after he received the recommendation, first said nothing and then, five weeks later, referred the issue to the Justice Department for further "review".

The President's delaying tactics are not the worst of the government's sins. As mentioned earlier, the federal government itself discriminates against people with HIV infection. There are questions about the legality of the federal government's conduct; its Job Corps policy has already been challenged in federal court, in part on constitutional grounds. But federal discrimination persists, and serves by example to undermine any arguments against discrimination by others.

Unlike the federal government, many of the state governments have worked forthrightly to curtail discrimination related to AIDS, by enacting new laws or by interpreting existing statutes expansively. In 1986, California passed a law prohibiting employers and insurance companies from requiring the HIV antibody test. New York's Division of Human Rights has made clear that it believes the state's "disability" discrimination statute covers AIDS, and the New York State Legislature recently enacted a law generally barring disclosure of HIV test results without the permission of the subject.

Private groups have also fought AIDS-related discrimination. In 1983, Lambda Legal Defense and Education Fund, an organization promoting civil rights for gay people, brought the first AIDS discrimination lawsuit in the United States. In that case, Lambda prevented the eviction of a doctor from his office because he treated patients with AIDS. The successful legal precedent of that case has led to similar results in other courts across the country. The Citizens Commission on AIDS for New York City and Northern New Jersey, created in 1986 by fifteen private foundations, drew up a set of principles on AIDS in the workplace based on the concept of equitable treatment, and then set about obtaining endorsements from employers. As of December 1988, more than three hundred had lent their names to the commission's guidelines.

Fear of AIDS, often accompanied by misunderstanding, continues to foster discrimination against people associated with AIDS, even those who are not at all sick or infected. The attention of the state governments and of some not-for-profit groups has helped somewhat to check discrimination, but, as James D. Watkins has observed, federal inattention seriously limits the success of their efforts.

From this assessment of AIDS in the United States, two major themes emerge. The first and most powerful is the extraordinary lethargy of the United States government. At best, the government has been negligent. At worst, it has actually made the epidemic worse, standing in the way of forces and developments that might prove beneficial. The government need not have taken on all the tasks itself, but it should have at least planned, advised, and coordinated. This it has not done although the cost to it of devising a preliminary national strategy on AIDS would have been insignificant in an annual federal budget of $1 trillion.

Why has the government been so irresponsible? The answer must be more than financial, for fiscal concerns, if taken seriously, generally militate for rather than against planning. This is especially true with AIDS: a truly effective prevention campaign now would substantially reduce future medical costs.

The explanation lies not in money but in politics. The populations most deeply affected by AIDS are outside the American mainstream: gay men, and intravenous drug users and their sexual partners and children, who are largely black or Hispanic. They have few political representatives, and few advocates. They, and the lives they lead, are viewed with distaste and disapproval by many Americans. Some Americans even see people with AIDS as willing and culpable victims. In a national survey published in 1987, more than one third of the respondents agreed with the statement "AIDS is God's punishment." James J. Kilpatrick, a well-known national newspaper columnist, wrote in June 1988: "My thought is that AIDS victims deserve about the same 'compassion' that society extends to those who smoke themselves to death or drink themselves to death." Sentiments of this sort, usually coupled with the notion that AIDS does not attack "normal" people, have sidetracked the calls for action of the President's Commission and the experts on AIDS. They have also severely distorted the public debate on AIDS, confusing the issue with a variety of other concerns only vaguely related to the epidemic itself.

Official neglect is not, however, the sole theme to emerge over the first seven years of the epidemic. There is a brighter one. In the face of governmental indifference, hundreds of thousands of Americans, some acting on their own behalf, others for the benefit of relatives, friends, colleagues, or neighbours, have joined together to furnish the services not available from the government. In less than a decade, they have fashioned an alternative and unofficial national network relying principally on volunteer labour. They have also collected many millions of dollars to sustain their efforts.

With adequate support from the federal government, the private organizations that fight AIDS could have done more. Nonetheless, their growth and accomplishments tell a lesson: non-government organizations should have a major part in any effective national strategy against AIDS. Such organizations permit greater diversity and experimentation. They absorb changes in approach more rapidly than is ordinarily possible for government bureaucracies. They also give communities and populations more voice in the shaping of solutions. All in all, privately-run organizations shorten the distance between those who serve and those who are served. Most gay men do take seriously advice from Gay Men's Health Crisis, or its companion organizations across the United States. Similarly, drug users may not listen to the Surgeon General or to the Secretary of Health and Human Services, but they do heed a former user employed as a counsellor by a local organization.

Two lessons emerge from the polarity between government inaction and private initiative. One concerns politics. AIDS is unlike any other public health issue. In each individual and in the body politic, it spurs sentiments that are likely to interfere with rational resolution of the crisis. AIDS requires special political leaders who will put public health concerns first, who will not shy from controversy, and who will step forward to mould and inform public opinion. The second relates to the scope of government action. No government should attempt to confront the crisis entirely by itself, even if it possesses the necessary will and resources. Private citizens, and private organizations, can often reach those in need more quickly and more effectively than government agencies. Government should foster the development of these independent efforts with, among other things, money and advice.

May other countries be guided, not by the sad example of the United States Government, but by the ingenuity and compassion of those US citizens who have taken it upon themselves to confront AIDS.

appear that all these groups have perhaps enabled the government both to starve AIDS funding and to distance itself from education work, research, and the care of people with AIDS.

One example which seems particularly pertinent concerns the early establishment of the National AIDS Trust. In 1987 the Minister of Health, Norman Fowler, called together representatives from the Terrence Higgins Trust, Body Positive, CRUSAID, the Department of Health and Social Security (DHSS) AIDS Unit, the Chief Medical Officer (CMO), and the Health Minister for discussion of the establishment of the National AIDS Trust. The overt agenda of this meeting was to co-ordinate the many services that were developing, and formulate an effective national plan for dealing with AIDS.

The hidden agenda of this meeting was how the Government could get away with spending as little as possible. It was quite clear that the Government wanted to get as much money from the community as it possibly could in order to reduce its own level of funding. It was also clear that it wanted to keep itself as far away as possible from any closely targeted education towards gay men and drug users. This remains manifest in the Health Education Authority adverts concerning the risk of AIDS to heterosexuals; there is no clearly targeted campaign for the gay community, whilst drug users are simply told "don't take drugs because it might give you AIDS".

Instead of getting up and banging the table at those meetings as we should have done, instead of pulling the rug from under the Government, we said: "Yes, we must do something. We must strengthen the voluntary sector. Yes we will do all we can to work with you." We willingly agreed that such funding as the Government might provide would go into education for gay men and drug users, but avoiding any direct association between them and the DHSS. The situation now facing us is extremely grim. The work that the gay community has done in fighting Section 28 of the 1988 Local Government Act has not been paralleled by any kind of direct challenge to the inadequacies of AIDS funding and Government policies. The breakdown of social service provision, the erosion of local government, the funding crisis of the National Health Service: all of these have a direct bearing on our needs as a community facing the problem of AIDS, both in education and research, as well as in the field of direct caring. Yet the Terrence Higgins Trust and other voluntary sector organizations have, with rare exceptions, singularly failed to grasp the need to put AIDS in its wider political context, to be prepared to fight for our basic requirements and rights. This would involve developing coherent strategies for revitalizing the NHS, and seeking a statutory guarantee of local government social service provision.

Instead, our immediate response to the tragedy of AIDS has been to rush off to hold people's hands at bedsides. We have not taken our fight out onto the streets as has happened in the United States. We have a great deal to learn from the 1987 March on Washington, and other directly political campaigns such as ACT UP. If at the very beginning of the crisis we had been able to align ourselves more closely with trades union activity and with the struggles in the NHS, we might not now be seen as a "special category" requiring separate hospices and services. We have been forced to resort to a kind of gay freemasonry in order to get action on vital issues such as housing, which should be a fundamental right.

When a very sick person needed housing or social service support, we did not feel we should make a "case" out of it. Perhaps we didn't have time, or it wasn't our choice to make. We achieved our immediate ends by harassing quiet gay men and women in positions of authority — the ones who didn't want to "make too much of a fuss", but still had a conscience. Looking back, I recognize that we should have tried to forge a broad base of support. Not just with other gay people, or those involved in drug-related work, but across the entire spectrum of British politics. We relied on community contacts, and on the sympathy of individuals, but we had not taken in the fact that AIDS requires a coherent political analysis.

An example from the London borough of Hammersmith and Fulham where I live: my lover George, who has AIDS, and I were recently rehoused. We were unceremoniously dumped in a house with absolutely no services — not even light bulbs in the sockets. The only way in which I managed to get any support whatsoever was because the emergency housing officers, whom I happened to know, were very concerned, and did all they could to help. One actually went so far as to take carpeting from his own home to give us something to cover the floor. In desperation I accepted this. In desperation we accept many things. We did have one visit from a social worker, who sat at the opposite end of the room when talking to George, refusing to come anywhere near his bed. I didn't fight that either at the time because we were only too grateful for whatever help we could get.

Unfortunately this has been a recurring theme in the history of social service provision up till now. Overwhelmed by the tragedy and crisis of dealing with AIDS, and overwhelmed by the pain of those whom we are counselling, we have attended to individual needs in an ad hoc manner, as best we can. But at the same time we should also have been mustering support and working to put AIDS firmly on the political agenda. And in that we have so far failed. We have seen what can be done in terms of concerted organization in the face of Section 28. If it is not yet too late, we must make sure that organizations working with AIDS stop gratefully thanking the government for its pathetic financial handouts and stop going to meetings behind closed doors saying to ourselves: "Well, this is *real* politics — this is how it is. Yes we will talk to Conservative politicians. Yes we do accept that you don't want to get your hands dirty by putting out explicit AIDS information for gay men and drug users, talking about sex and condoms. Yes, we'll do your job for you." But we should *not* be prepared to cover up for the Government, and to do its job for it. We must insist that we are as much a part of the body politic as anybody else. We have a right to expect the same services that any other community expects — even if these are not necessarily forthcoming these days. We are going to have to become more political. We are going to have to take to the streets to protest against the cutbacks in the NHS and the crippling of local government, because, as people affected by AIDS, we are *part* of those struggles.

Until we are able to bring about a new awareness in the voluntary sector and stop being more or less willing accomplices to the increasing marginalization of people with HIV and ARC and AIDS, these problems are likely to become far worse. It is simply not enough that organizations such as the Terrence Higgins Trust should get more money. It is not enough that we open hospices such as the London Lighthouse. We have to force government, and other institutions such as the press and TV, to understand what we actually have to *do* in our work for and on behalf of people with AIDS. I am reminded of a story I heard concerning a woman facing cancer on her own. I could identify with her problems, which had little to do with gender and nothing to do with sexuality. The challenges she was faced with arose directly from the inadequacy of social services and the erosion of local government and the NHS. These are the very problems that confront my lover and myself every day.

Whilst it is far from clear that we will succeed in preventing ourselves from being further marginalized, and uniting what are sometimes seen as different and distinct areas of struggle, we must certainly start to consider AIDS in terms of a perspective of the centralization of political power and the decimation of local government in the UK today. If one considers a case like Manchester, where real progress has been made in the fight against AIDS on a genuine community basis, or the example of the Greater London Council before its abolition, one quickly realizes how terribly damaging the erosion of local government has been.

Such thoughts are very painful. I and my colleagues in the voluntary sector have struggled long and hard in the course of the past five years. It hurts to question if the focus of our work was mistaken. But none of us had the wisdom of hindsight, nor the long experience of government and its many agencies that we now possess. Looking forwards, we have to demand that the needs of people with AIDS are acknowledged as a basic humanitarian issue in a "civilized" society. We must insist that the gay community should not always have to lead the fight against AIDS, on top of trying to cope with all our individual and collective experience of grief and loss. Yet the fight against AIDS has also been a crucible, in which many, many people have been strengthened and empowered — not least people with AIDS themselves. Our achievements in the years to come depend on just how successfully we can communicate the experiences of the past five years, both good and bad, to those now entering the fray.

This is a revised version of the talk given at the ICA conference.

CINDY PATTON

THE AIDS INDUSTRY

Construction of "Victims", "Volunteers" and "Experts"

We are experiencing a dawning recognition that while science
constructs our reality, it cannot save us from our human limitations.
This is made clear by current cultural and political responses to AIDS,
which are at once a throwback to medieval notions of sin and
disease, and a confrontation with a cybernetic future of slow viruses
and technologized sex.

In the Age of Reason, the feudal and clerical orders of human
difference were recast through the construction of modern
taxonomies of science. Today, information control — which has as
dubious a claim as science to objectivity — has been mobilized to
reorganize categories of class, race and sexuality in accordance with
the unreason that characterizes responses to AIDS. Initiated from
different sectors of the media, scientific journals, and public policy
journals, the new ideas of class and sexuality are both contradictory
and contested: they produce ideological paradoxes and open up
strategic possibilities for resisting the racism, classism, sexism and
homophobia written into the AIDS crisis.

I became interested in the reorganization of race, class and
sexuality after seeing the homophobia and racism (less often,
sexism and classism) that seem to prevent natural allies in the fight
against AIDS from working together. As AIDS developed as a political
and social crisis, I became perplexed by the continued inability of
gay community groups to work with leaders and organizations from
communities of colour, despite their stated good intentions. The
sense of urgency and the obvious benefits of working together
could surely have outweighed the historic stumbling blocks

between these communities both nationally and locally. The recent inclusion of lesbians and gay men in the Rainbow Coalition and the greater mutual understanding forged over years of progressive organizing might be seen to have laid the groundwork for cooperation around AIDS. There is, however, an emerging hegemony of AIDS groups; a hierarchy that signals a broader problem than local histories or poorly planned strategies could account for. In looking at the way AIDS service and education are provided in the late 1980s, I began to understand what I will call the "AIDS industry" as having institutionalized a pattern of racism, sexism, and classism, while it struggles to stave off queer-baiting.

I have chosen the idea of an AIDS industry —which I understand roughly as the combination of public health service and private-sector non-profit organizations devoted exclusively to AIDS work —because it implies a set of social relations based on shared norms, styles of organizational behaviour, and institutionalized thought patterns, rather than a collusion of the powerful who maintain an "establishment" by coercion, or who simply function as a money-making centre. The notion of an "industry" is of course in some sense a fiction, and runs the danger of over-generalizing and obscuring local experience. Nevertheless, there is value in identifying the hidden policy assumptions and material conditions that construct AIDS as a "particular" type of problem and legitimate "particular" solutions. It is important to differentiate between the industry, with its rules and norms, and the people involved as staff or volunteers in such groups. Individuals will have a wide range of views of their role in such organizations, and may feel conflicts with the internal or external aims and objectives of the industry. Understanding them as working within an "industry" is, however, useful, in that it serves to uncover the full implications of homophobia, racism, classism and sexism in the handling of AIDS in particular communities or groups.

From Grassroots to Business Suits

There was a major shift in the fight against AIDS between mid 1985 and mid 1986 in the largest US cities. This shift was away from gay resistance to a hostile government and indifferent medical empire, and toward an assimilation of activists into a new AIDS industry, with its own set of commitments, its own structuring logic. This shift occurred in part because the gay community was gaining the power of self-determination in AIDS work on a gay liberation agenda, and there was concern that other minority groups might also lay claim to power on counter-cultural agendas. 1985 saw the end of the media blackout, which had permitted only a handful of sensational or overly medical articles to be printed. 1985 also saw the first wave of public awareness that AIDS was affecting heterosexuals who were neither transfusion recipients nor IV-drug users. For a brief time in 1985 — as government agencies surveyed what had been done, and what was to be done — the large gay AIDS organizations were perceived as expert because of their experience with AIDS over the previous few years. But as government and media interest increased, it became common to hear that gay men were a special "lobby", rather than "experts". As gay community-based AIDS groups worked more and more with the government, they spoke less directly of sex, and government officials — at least in the more liberal state and local governments — learned not to make embarrassing homophobic remarks. But this decreasing discussion of homosexuality was not, as the large AIDS groups argued, a result of decreased homophobia. Indeed, the right considered this "de-gaying" of the AIDS debate to be a plot to obscure the "real truth" about AIDS. The de-gaying of AIDS discourse was simultaneous with a heightening of class and race anxieties around AIDS, and we must measure decreases in homophobia against increases of racism and classism in this new AIDS industry.

By 1986, the major AIDS organizations had been socialized into, and become vehicles for socializing people into, a new paradigm —a new understanding of the meaning and organization of AIDS which radically separated the groups from their liberationist roots. The AIDS groups closed ranks with government agencies, even while holding the line on mandatory testing, discrimination, and related policy issues. The emergence within AIDS groups of an identifiable professional style — of a commitment to professional standards and tests of efficacy — coincides with the first major influx of federal government funding for AIDS education and services, in late 1985. AIDS groups and government officials alike believed that AIDS cases would continue to be diagnosed at an alarming rate and that society at large would be financially and socially affected by the AIDS epidemic. In the face of widespread denial of AIDS, this shared perception reinforced the affinity between community groups and public health officials and diminished the real differences in their strategies. The AIDS groups realized they needed government funds, and government officials realized they needed the guidance and support as well as the huge volunteer base of the AIDS groups.

But this new industry was not content with this massive, if sometimes uneasy conjunction of money and people: it needed also to rewrite the history of the community response to AIDS in order to justify its methods of coping with the epidemic. In what follows, I shall be looking at how the industry's image of itself demanded the construction of a new AIDS narrative, with "victims", "experts" and "volunteers" as its dramatis personae.[1] An assessment of the industry's covert policy bias may be unearthed by asking three questions: who controls information? who gets the message? and who gets care? The white, middle-class dominated AIDS industry in the US — and the Western-dominated AIDS agencies worldwide — not only control funds, but determine who is allowed to speak about AIDS.

Who Controls Information?

Control over AIDS information in the past two to three years has been simultaneously professionalized and democratized through a series of contradictory processes, three of which I shall discuss here: the introduction of "media AIDS experts", the institution of alternative HIV antibody test sites (ATS), and the introduction of traditionally trained health education professionals. These new hierarchies of power control the production and targeting of AIDS information.

The emergence of media experts has increased the gap between the producers and consumers of scientific knowledge. Media translators fall prey to elisions and simplifications: their use of terms such as "the AIDS test"[2], "promiscuity", "AIDS carrier" distorts the scientific facts and their social implications. Media science articulates the same old prejudices in a new "objective" language: science reporters pretend that gay activists and right-wing fanatics have "politicized" AIDS, yet do not acknowledge the political implications of the way the media carves out the AIDS information landscape.

Second, there is non-diagnostic HIV antibody testing, which is widely seen to have democratized AIDS education in the face of impenetrable "facts" about exotic viruses and amazing new drugs. The so-called alternative test sites, funded and supervised through state and federal programmes, were established in late 1985, after the antibody test had become available that spring. They were called "alternative", not in the leftist or progressive sense, but because they represented an "alternative" to seeking knowledge of HIV antibody status through blood donation.[3]

The alternative test sites have since emerged as the centre for socializing individuals (as opposed to communities) to the new reality of HIV. The media and government-funded AIDS education programmes promote HIV antibody testing as the centrepiece of their campaign to stop AIDS. The belief of many policy makers that it is widespread testing and not community organizing that has slowed the spread of HIV among gay men, has made plausible such bills as the Helm's Amendment in the US and Section 28 of the Local Government Act in Britain. The passage of these ultra-homophobic laws stems directly from a denial of the role of positive gay identity in risk assessment and the reduction of HIV transmission. The public health debate in the US pretends that "neutral" testing can solve the problem, although nearly every other country in the world rejects widespread testing programmes as expensive, ineffective, and misleading as an educational strategy.[4]

Non-diagnostic uses of the HIV antibody test promote the construction of a sexual identity based on perceived risk and test result. In the early years of the epidemic, community efforts were focused on replacing the notion of risk *groups* — homosexuals, IV-drug users, prostitutes, partners of all the above — with that of risk *behaviour*, which includes sharing unclean needles, and engaging in intercourse without a condom. Testing has simply revised the risk categories to "positive" and "negative"; no regard is paid to the significant mislabeling induced by testing error. The implicit association between positivity and high risk behaviour, negativity and purity fail to dissolve the stigma and patterns of discrimination already insinuated into AIDS risk logic: the "risky behaviour" for which testing is essentially a confirmatory exercise is already associated in the public mind with gay men, prostitutes, drug users, and people of colour.

Finally, the introduction of health education professionals to a pre-existing AIDS and safe sex education framework brought a different attitude toward reducing the incidence of AIDS. Professional health educators demanded empirical rather than experiential proof that particular strategies worked. Their behaviourist orientation blinded them to the symbolic meanings and social organization of both sex and IV-drug use: they failed to recognize that the people they sought to educate pursued their pleasures in communities and subcultures that operated by rules different from those of main-stream society. Health education professionals trained in the "scared straight" style of education manipulated existing fears, making it difficult to separate false, pedagogically-inspired panic from real causes of alarm. Overly individualistic in their approach, the professionals never realized that gay men and IV-drug users had coped with the fear and reality of AIDS long before they arrived on the scene. But, both subcultures had already begun to adapt to new group mores promoting safer practices and had begun a defence against the repression accompanying the AIDS epidemic.

Safer practices brought increased social attack. For IV-drug users, getting one's own needles meant risking arrest for carrying. For gay men, promoting condom use meant publicly highlighting the practice of anal sex, a great social taboo in the US. Nevertheless, there had been a significant reduction in sexual risk among gay men by 1985 — three years before professional educators exerted influence in the burgeoning AIDS industry. These shifts in mores — enough to reduce sero-conversion in San Francisco to less than 2 per cent per year in 1987 — were made by activists with little knowledge of traditional health education theory or strategy.[5]

Safe Sex: Who Gets the Message?
Safe sex organizing efforts before 1985 grew out of the gay community's understanding of the social organization of our own sexuality and from extrapolations of information hidden in epidemiologic studies. Informed by a self-help model taken from the women's health movement and by the gay liberation discussion of sexuality, safe sex was viewed by early AIDS activists, not merely as a practice to be imposed on the reluctant, but as a form of political resistance and community building that achieved both sexual liberation and sexual health. It was this liberatory subtext that seems to have most raised the ire of the far right, and it was the first premiss of safe sex organizing to be lost when professionals unveiled their plans for safer sex education.

The first safe sex advice created by gay men was constructed in opposition to the dictates of doctors. By 1983, there was so much safe sex advice that a group of gay men, including men with AIDS wrote a 40-page booklet entitled *How to Have Sex in An Epidemic*. It still stands as the single most comprehensive guide to safe sex; it

includes explanations of theories of transmission, sexual techniques, and the psycho-social problems of coping with the change
to safe sex and with the fear of AIDS. It is important to realize that this
booklet was written *before* a virus was associated with AIDS: men
understood and made major, effective changes without the benefit
of HIV antibody testing. Scientific studies of transmission have not
changed the lists of safe and unsafe acts enumerated in the first safe
sex guidelines. If anything, HIV has proved *more* difficult to transmit
than was at first suspected, and infection thus more solidly linked to
that sharing of unclean needles, the introduction of semen into the
rectum and vagina, and the use of unscreened blood products. Yet
the professional health educators who have dominated the field
since 1985–86 would have people believe that a personal safe sex
plan based on a few facts and a lot of common sense is always
ineffective. Professional health educators displace the authority for
understanding and encouraging safe sex standards from those who
engage in sex, onto medical experts.

Despite their lack of involvement in AIDS work before 1985–86,
health education professionals have claimed the credit for the
community-wide shifts in mores represented by the San Francisco
sero-conversion statistics. They play on this success to promote their
own, traditional, "scared straight" style of education — as one friend
of mine in state government said, "Syphilis didn't work, herpes
didn't work, but AIDS works."[6]

Professional educators have ignored or let atrophy the more
innovative grassroots programmes — such as those that trained
bar-tenders as educators, or a community-involvement project of
zap actions, where leather-clad hunks raided bars to pass out
condoms and AIDS literature. Mr Leather, a gay man chosen through a
"leather" contest, is still mandated by the organizations that support
him to spend his year doing safe sex education. Last year's Miss
America also wanted to do AIDS education; she was prevented on the
grounds that it would be considered unbecoming. Most educators
today are no longer willing to take social risks in order to promote
sexual safety. This rationalist pedagogy sets up a system of
categories which make those who do not "hear the message"
subject to special emergency measures and laws. Professionalized
AIDS education tends to direct programmes at good learners, not at
those who most need concrete, non-judgmental information and
support for making changes in their lives. Evaluation techniques

like pre- and post-testing of information, and charting sero-conversion levels within communities, do not adequately reflect the types and levels of real changes in groups that are subject to the pressures of poverty and policing, or which have differing self-conceptions of risk, safety, and the value of the community versus the individual. The CDC (Centers for Disease Control: the US agency that tracks AIDS and HIV and sponsors much of the education) requires a testing component in most educational programmes it funds, not only because it believes testing reinforces behaviour change, but because testing allows access to communities where consent to education programmes would not otherwise be given.

A number of the communities most directly affected by AIDS and HIV infection are, then, seriously disenfranchised by the white middle-class style and pedagogy of the AIDS industry. Yet in communities of colour, among IV-drug users, among prostitutes and in several African nations, exciting projects in AIDS education are underway. These projects demand community involvement, are open-ended, and rely on the idea that the *process* of AIDS education is important in determining how AIDS is perceived and whether behaviour changes are effected. These programmes are now well funded, and are in danger of professionalization and absorption just like projects by and for the gay male community.

Who Gets Care? The New Altruism

Like health education, care for people with AIDS in the US duplicates existing, unequal structures of delivery of health care, consolidating class and race divisions. Poor people with HIV related ailments are cared for — if they get an AIDS related diagnosis at all — in city hospitals or by their family in the home; or they end up in shelters or on the street. While the major AIDS organizations have created group homes for homeless people with AIDS, they have difficulty in reaching and working with people who were already in poverty before their AIDS related illness.

When people with AIDS are taken care of at home, the result is exhausted relatives, friends, or young children who have to provide food, clean and help the person with AIDS every minute of the day. Though these are unpaid services, these poor, often black or Latin relatives and friends are not the people identified within the AIDS industry as "volunteers". Even in the middle-class gay male community, the work of friends is differentiated from the work of volunteers who are predominantly gay men and straight women from the white middle class.

The AIDS groups that now call such people volunteers began as grassroots organizations with liberationist ideology. AIDS activists worked with PWA's in the context of community organizing rather than altruism. Their grassroots ideology fostered identification with PWA's and with the gay community; thus lesbians, for example, became involved, not because they were personally at risk, but because they were part of a community under assault. This sense of community resistance created the possibility of forming coalitions with communities of colour which were being silently ravaged by AIDS and the AIDS related backlash.

However, this remains largely unrealized. By 1986, AIDS had become an acceptable vehicle for the new altruism promoted by Reaganism. Under President Reagan, federal funding of most social service programmes was cut, and state and local government private foundations were asked to pick up the bill. This was supposed to be more cost efficient, and to instil traditional values like charity and gratitude in both "volunteers" and "victims". In reality, it meant those with the time took care of their own. While the black community tightened its ranks through its social agencies and churches, the predominantly white, gay non-profit AIDS agencies tacitly regrouped around race and class allegiances. The media valorized the gay male volunteer who put aside his career and personal fears of AIDS to care for his brothers. Straight white women also volunteered in large numbers, not because they were at risk of HIV infection through their boyfriends or husbands, but because they are the traditional volunteer reservoir. Many were personally affected by gay male friends with AIDS, but they were not encouraged to look at this experience in their social context, nor to challenge the sexism they encountered in the division of labour and the ideology of the AIDS industry. This influx of women was taken as a sign that the white middle class was educated about AIDS and had overcome its homophobia. Yet straight white men are almost never AIDS volunteers — unless they are part of the haemophiliac community or have a close relative with AIDS. But they do earn their salaries in the AIDS industry; they are the researchers, administrators, journalists — the experts, the neutral professionals who are above politics and frequently have no contact with people in the communities most harshly affected by AIDS.

Why, suddenly in 1985–86, when people still feared casual contact, did white middle-class men allow their wives and sisters to get involved in AIDS groups? That these women should be perceived as safe from gay men stems from the long and special relationship between straight white women and their faggot hairdresser or designer, a relationship that reinforces sexual and gender norms by putting women under the supervision of "non-threatening" men during their leisure time. AIDS might have broken this persistent link — already somewhat displaced by feminist and gay liberationist critiques of gender roles. Instead, these two stereotypes were reinforced, in a set of manoeuvres that acted to consolidate class and male power.

Thus Reagan's new altruism has diffused the political power of community organizing, by recasting as "good works" middle-class efforts to help itself in the face of federal funding cuts in social programmes. It ends any society-wide commitment to redistributing wealth, and instead allocates resources according to who makes appealing "victims".[7] It even rationalizes the funding cuts by making the middle-class volunteer a model: "see what the faggots have done for themselves with no government money?" Implicitly, the black community is called upon to do likewise.

The Price of Organizational Amnesia
Why was there such a need to direct community organizing into non-profit altruism? The gay community and to a lesser extent IV-drug subculture were already successful in changing their group patterns to reduce the risk of HIV transmission. These changes were accomplished through a self-empowerment model within highly articulated sexual and drug cultures, by building rather than dismantling communities. Safe sex and safe drug use campaigns consolidated these communities, highlighting the ways in which the existing organization of sex and drug use was influenced by the anti-sex, anti-drug, anti-pleasure ideology of the dominant US culture. This community organizing effort made it clear that AIDS was a product of medical neglect, and of the legal oppression of gay men and drug users. The experience of coping with AIDS within these communities was highly politicizing in the early years — and

remains so for people who refuse to adopt the expert/volunteer/victim categories.

Today, a growing number of white AIDS activists, and the communities of colour in general, view the major AIDS organizations as indistinguishable from government agencies, or agencies directed toward less controversial diseases. AIDS groups are now largely dominated by white, middle-class values and staffed by gay male and straight female volunteers.[8] Satisfied in the belief that they have overcome their middle-class homophobia, they now direct education toward those most likely to accept the middle-class view of AIDS as simply a tragic disease, which has been made a political issue by noisy gays and right-wing crazies. Educational and direct-service projects are built on a middle-class model and offered to anyone who will accept that model. Less time and effort goes into developing new models because those who reject the efforts of these AIDS groups are seen as intransigent, not as potential allies in a coalition seeking self-determination and the just apportioning of medical care and social services. The new altruism divides those in need of services into the grateful and ungrateful, marginalizing those who, because of their past and current experience of medical care, are demanding radical change. In the end, the voice of those most affected by AIDS has no purchase against the paradigms of the "expert"; while "volunteers" are becoming voiceless collaborators in the narrow range of programmes that are being developed by the new AIDS industry.

Notes

1.The terms in quotes are not intended to indicate how people with AIDS, AIDS activists, medical workers, or others may refer to themselves. Indeed much energy has been spent since the beginning of the epidemic to stop people from referring to people with AIDS, ARC, or HIV infection as "victims" or "sufferers". When I use the term "victim", I mean to say that the industry, whatever rubric it uses for its objects — clients, people with AIDS, the acronym PWA — essentially considers them as "victims", unable to speak for or about themselves, unable to suggest policy because of their status. Similarly, "volunteer" is a special category used to refer to people who have received the appropriate training/indoctrination and work with "victims" in the proper fashion, with the proper emotional attitude. They are not helpful policy makers, because they are too close to the "victims" and are assumed to be acting out of pure motives, not political ones. Only the "experts", who themselves may be members of "high-risk" communities, are allowed to suggest policy, and then only through the proper channels and with the proper pedagogy and view of what AIDS service means.

2. The widely offered test is, technically, a test for antibodies to Human Immunodeficiency Virus (HIV), the virus generally believed to render the immune system incapable of fighting the relatively common opportunistic infections which become fatal in AIDS. The test, which has both high false positive and false negative rates, does not tell who will progress to clinical AIDS, or show who will manifest any symptoms. The correlation between infection and antibody status is unknown. Time between infection with virus and production of antibodies can be anywhere between six weeks and eighteen months.

3. The HIV antibody test was initially designed for screening blood donations. Before a virus was identified and a screening test available, blood banks asked donors at high risk to refrain from donating. A check list and pamphlet were given to donors, who were expected to assess their risk or ask questions. Blood banks agreed that voluntary donor deferral was highly successful and screening would further reduce donation of blood by people who didn't realize or understand their risk. Gay activists argued that blood testing positive — which included a large number of false positive units — should be destroyed but that donors should not be put on any register that might open them to discrimination. Blood banks finally rejected this idea and decided that they had a moral obligation and legal liability to notify those whose blood was rejected that they had tested postive for HIV antibody and should seek additional counselling or medical advice. The blood banks then feared that, if it became widely known that testing was available at donation sites, high-risk people might come in for testing and HIV infected units might slip by undetected, since there is also a small but significant number of false negative tests. Thus, the decision to notify donors of their test result meant that donating might be used for self-testing. It was this fear, apparently, that led to the creation of sites where anonymous testing could take place. These were the so-called alternative test sites.

4. The exceptions are West Germany, Japan, Cuba, and South Africa, where there is testing. Sweden has a highly coercive testing policy and the tabloid press in Britain as well as the fascist National Front advocate mass testing.

5. Since it takes between six weeks and eighteen months from infection to production of antibody — sero-conversion — a 2 per cent rate in early 1987 means that significant changes had already taken place in the years before. The sero-conversion rates for HIV must be taken in this long view, unlike rates for syphilis or gonorrhoea, which reflect infections in the previous few weeks or months.

6. Some AIDS workers in San Francisco say they believe the community has been given credit for accomplishing this work. The opinions about testing, studies of the role of testing in behaviour change, and fear about abuse of testing are quite different in San Francisco from elsewhere in the US. In general, community leaders and AIDS activists seem to feel comfortable with existing confidentiality procedures, and studies from the densely gay areas of San Francisco indicate that test knowledge seems to reinforce behaviour change. However, virtually identical studies conducted among gay men in Baltimore and Chicago, and different studies in New York City among gay men and IV-drug users do not show a correlation between test knowledge and shifts toward safer sex techniques.

7. In New York city, for example, Gay Men's Health Crisis (GMHC) has a $10 million budget and a staff of about seventy-five, while the Minority AIDS Task Force (MATF) has a budget of $1 million, and a staff of eight. Half the cases of AIDS in New York City are people of colour.

8. It is difficult to get sexual orientation breakdowns of female volunteers, but discussions with AIDS organizers from the US, Australia, Britain, and Canada suggest that while there may be some lesbians working in the major AIDS groups, those with political commitments to self-help feel alienated in these groups. At least some of these lesbians have begun autonomous organizing around women-with-AIDS issues and around prostitutes. The fact that prostitutes and poor women, major objects of concern for female altruists at the turn of the century, have not been deemed good "victims" by the AIDS industry can probably be attributed to the sexism that prevents women volunteers from setting organizational agendas. That straight women have not pressed their gay male comrades to direct safe sex education at straight men is equally suggestive of sexism.

First of all, I think it is very important to understand the political milieu in which the AIDS crisis has developed in Great Britain, as in America. Central to this (absolutely central, in my opinion) is the agenda setting of the last decade by the New Right — agenda setting on a whole host of social and cultural issues but in particular, as we're beginning to experience more forcefully in Britain since the 1987 general election, agenda setting in terms of the sexual behaviour of all of us. This has gone hand-in-hand with what to some extent has been the continuing liberalization of attitudes towards sexuality during the past decade on all the measures of public opinion in relationship to most forms of sexual behaviour. But over the past two or three years, as recent evidence has shown, there has been a shuddering setback in public attitudes towards homosexuality — a very significant drop, for instance, of about 20 per cent of those polled, who are in favour of continuing liberalization of the law. This is very significant, and is obviously very closely related to the AIDS crisis. What I want to suggest, though, is that this is not simply the development of homophobia. There is certainly a deep, entrenched fear and hostility towards homosexuality but I don't think what's happened in relationship to, say, Section 28 of the Local Government Act (which bans local authorities from "promoting" homosexuality) can simply be understood in terms of a mobilization of homophobia.

The first thing I want to say about the British New Right, which I think is very interestingly different from its American counterpart, is that its roots are not in a fundamentalist religious tradition. The roots of the New Right in this country are much more explicitly political. It is very interesting, for instance, that it is only in 1987/88, after something like ten years of agenda setting by the New Right in Britain, that we have the Church of England agonizing over how to deal with homosexuality. In the United States, debates on the nature of sexual behaviour began before it was politically appropriated. In this country, the political appropriation of these issues by the New Right, precedes any important religious preoccupation. This is very significant and is the reason why the backlash against homosexuality in particular has become more organized in this country than in the United States. And the reason I stress this is because it is not simply homophobia that the New Right is articulating. It is more a positive agenda than a negative reaction to the so-called permissiveness of the 1960s, a positive agenda in terms of the reinstatement of "the family" and family values.

The Government's action over Section 28 is very much a by-product of that attempt to reassert familial values. This is quite clear in the actual framing of the legislation. There was obviously an element of political opportunism behind the Government's action, the desire to take advantage of the backlash against what many Labour local authorities had done since the mid 1980s. There had also been a half decade of antagonistic reporting by the tabloids in relationship to homosexuality and AIDS. But much more than that, Section 28 was an opportunity to reaffirm the importance of family values. The phrasing of the legislation itself is very indicative: it prohibits local authorities from promoting homosexuality as a "pretended family relationship". This is the key to what is happening sexually: it is actually an attempt to stop the formal recognition of homosexuality as on a par with heterosexuality.

That is important in itself, but of course it is also important in terms of response to the AIDS crisis. The Government found itself in a slight knot on this, and in Section 28 explicitly disconnects its ban on the promotion of homosexuality from education on AIDS. Here, as elsewhere, the Thatcher Government's ideological commitments become entangled with its pragmatic needs to contain a major health crisis.

This brings me to a second point which is equally important and that is the fact that the health crisis around AIDS and HIV coincides with a much more generalized crisis around the health service. I was very struck a couple of years ago when I was at a conference on AIDS in Sweden by a difference that emerged in the papers between those who had been brought up in the American tradition and those who came from a much more social-democratic, European and Australasian tradition. An interesting dichotomy developed between the Americans who stressed the importance of voluntary work and of self-activity, and the Swedes who stressed the importance of the role of the state in dealing with the health crisis. Those of us from Britain were somewhere in between in this debate, stressing the importance of voluntary activity but also the role of the state.

I was struck by Cindy Patton's querying of "professionalization", and her critique of an AIDS industry based on the "new altruism". This jolts with me, because the Anglo-Saxon tradition, which I think is an important tradition, stresses the importance of altruism in social policy and it is not something that can be simply written out of our response to the AIDS crisis. In particular the health service in this country is the embodiment of our spirit of altruism; and it is of critical importance that despite all the political and moral shifts that have taken place during the 1980s, this is still the one bastion of the social-democratic tradition that the Thatcher Government is finding very difficult to undermine.

This leads me to a third point: the needs of the different communities that are affected by AIDS. The Government partially recognizes the different needs of different communities, or at least the fact of different communities, in the targeting of its advertisements in relationship to AIDS. But there is an important difference between America and Britain in relationship to the acceptance of the pluralization of society — the fact of the existence of diverse communities. The central difference is the presence in the United States of what we can call a discourse of rights — a belief that these communities have a right to self-organize and to create their own milieus and to claim recognition from the community at large — and the total absence in the UK of any similar discourse of rights.

Nevertheless, beneath the surface, there is a profound shift in the political and social geography of Britain which the right recognizes much better than the left. And that is the fact of the emergence of communities of choice, elective communities I prefer to call them, which have become the foci of individual identities and ways of life. The gay community is the most obvious one in the context of AIDS, though not the only relevant one. Whatever its weaknesses, the gay community is clearly now a profound element in the political situation, because what it does is to link a personal identity to a sense of common feeling and common action across the bounds of class and gender, whatever the tensions within the community around class, gender and race. The gay community is, of course, a different sort of community from the black communities, but the black communities and the gay communities, and other communities of choice that are emerging, pose tremendous political problems, particularly for the left. What is critical about them in relationship to AIDS is that all these different communities voice questions about sexuality, about family styles, about sexual choices, about sexual identities.

Now here the difference between the communities is important, because one of the crucial things about the gay community is that it has been explicitly organized around sexuality, which makes it easier for it to talk about sexuality in relationship to the AIDS crisis. Other communities are not so explicitly organized around sexual issues and therefore have been more reluctant to discuss issues about unsafe sexual practices and changing sexual behaviour and so on. But what this point underlines is the critical importance of the involvement of the communities in the process of education around sexuality and sexual change.

One of the responses of the Thatcher Government to the NHS crisis is very much to emphasize privatization; and this is likely to be the drift of the change over the next two or three years. Where better to privatize than those communities of choice, which are coherent and strong? But it is at this point that the rhetoric of privatization and the devolution of responsibility comes up hard against other tendencies within New Right thought which are hostile to these communities, which want to see a homogeneous British society where these communities don't exist as separate foci of identity. This is a critical contradiction in the whole drift of "Thatcherite" politics, one of its many contradictions, which stem in part from the tension that exists between, on the one hand, a sort of social authoritarianism and, on the other hand, economic liberalism. These two strands often co-habit in extreme tension. And that tension, I would add, is a point of contestation and intervention — not a point of despair.

The fourth point I want to make is about the balance between communities of choice and the community as a whole. The AIDS crisis demands the mobilization of massive resources which can only be organized through the state and its agencies. Now it is here that there is a bigger difference between America and the UK. The USA values voluntary effort to an extent that British traditions do not. I think it is right and a social duty in a just society that the resources of the community are used for all its citizens, in particular when dealing with a huge health crisis. But that poses the problem of what the appropriate relationship should be between communities of choice and the state; and this, it seems to me, is a profound problem for the left, one which has hardly been dealt with at all. It is an issue indeed that goes beyond particular political traditions. It is here that the question of professionalization and the "new altruism" comes in again. It is very important that we do criticize aspects of the "top-down" approach that professionalization can give rise to. But it is necessary to say two things on this. One, it seems to me that professionalization is not necessarily a bad thing. It is much better to do things well than to do things badly. Those of us who came through left and gay groups in the seventies were, I think, misled by the belief that we should all learn to do absolutely everything to show that the division of labour was an artificial construct. It is now important to affirm that the division of labour is a good thing if it produces better health care and better facilities generally. The second point I would stress is that altruism is an essential element in any just society and not something that one should fear or despise. The critical issue is how professionalization and altruism are negotiated and balanced. The real danger is not so much those two things per se, but a managerial ethic and a bureaucratization which replicates a top-down model. Against this model, I would want to stress the critical importance of thinking through the relationship between professionals and the various communities as a democratic, rather than inevitably a bureaucratic, relationship.

Notes

This is a revised version of the talk given at the ICA conference.

1. Frank Mort, *Dangerous Sexualities: Medico-Moral Politics in England Since 1830*, London 1987.
2. See pages 113 to 125 of this book.

health information on AIDS and how to avoid it. It had shown an obvious and grotesque disregard for the needs and interests of gay men. The gay men who were the first to die of AIDS in this country were neither warned nor mourned. But by 1986 the disease was known to be spreading into the heterosexual population in the US. The government health warnings we have seen have thus been primarily aimed at heterosexual men and designed above all else to elicit a general fear of sex, rather than any positive desire for safe and pleasurable sexual encounters.

The male-oriented and sexually repressive message of the official propaganda campaign around AIDS is troubling, if only because with these biases it is less likely to be effective. In Africa, where transmission is primarily heterosexual, it is women who are most active in designing and leading the campaigns to contain the AIDS epidemic which, due largely to inadequate medical resources, is likely to kill over one million people in the next ten years.[2] The first cases of AIDS appeared at the same time in Africa and the US (1980–81) and, like those in the West today, the early African education programmes were designed for and aimed at men. Their failure shifted the emphasis to women. Women's involvement in family planning, their concern for their children, their more responsible attitude towards health care and sexuality, made women the obvious agents for changing sexual practices.[3] If this shift is to be mirrored in the developed world — if it is women who will be most involved in combating the heterosexual spread of AIDS — should not a feminist voice at least be involved in setting the agenda?

It is clear already that within the heterosexual population in Britain it is women who are more worried about AIDS than men— despite their slow rate of infection so far. This is hardly surprising. Women, almost everywhere, have rarely been able find pleasure in sex with men unaware of its accompanying dangers— whether of pregnancy, venereal disease, the health risks of contraception or, increasingly for younger women, cervical cancer. So far few women in Britain have become HIV positive through sex with men, but in New York AIDS from heterosexual sex is becoming the largest single cause of death among young women. Nor is it suprising that it is women, and in particular feminists— along with gay men— who have been most prominent in fighting for changes in dominant sexual practices. The most enduring and significant of women's struggles has been the long battle for women's control of their own fertility and sexuality. Its goal was and is for women to be free to choose when and if to have a child and for women to obtain sexual pleasure free from fears of pregnancy, disease and male coercion. It is conspicuous, therefore that— with a few notable exceptions— AIDS has not been taken up as a feminist issue.[4]

There are a number of reasons for the weak and belated feminist response to AIDS. It is not just that many of us, like everyone else, were unaware until recently of the fast spread of the disease. It is also that many feminists today have found it difficult to distance themselves effectively from the popular and persistant mainstream reaction to AIDS, which is simply and straightforwardly anti-sex. Conservative sexual politics have always been with us. But they re-emerged with a new confidence and determination at the close of the seventies when, with the election of conservative governments in Britain, the US and elsewhere, we heard again from every side a re-assertion of traditional family values and authoritarian sexual ethics. It was a self-serving "morality", necessary to justify Tory cut-backs in state welfare expenditure and any notion of collective provision for people's needs. The onset of AIDS gave this pro-family, anti-sexual permissiveness rhetoric an apparent legitimacy, not simply in the name of conservative morality but also in the name of medical wisdom.

"On *doctor's* orders the holiday must end," wrote journalist Pearson Phillips, aged 59, heaving a sigh of relief on behalf of many a middle-aged swinger from the sixties in the *Mail on Sunday.* "AIDS: IS ALL THE HYSTERIA A BLESSING IS DISGUISE?" asked *Good Housekeeping* in November 1986, curiously echoing Mary Whitehouse's vengeful and vicious pronouncement on behalf of the crusaders of the moral right. "Yes," replied the once self-proclaimed "naughty" feminist Erica Jong, having stashed away the profits from her titillating best-sellers on adulterous sex. Perhaps, she speculates, wistfully recalling her adolescence in the fifties, "we are going back to a stricter morality now," which makes sex "a little more mysterious and precious again." (The precious mystery of the "fallen woman" and the backstreet abortion.) She even indulges a little populist socio-biology, reflecting on "our old animal natures . . . programmed to reproduce and to regard reproduction as the highest good."[5] The theme is echoed, if with less hypocrisy and confused biologism, by

American feminist Gloria Steinem in the *Observer*: "The sexual revolution is not our [women's] revolution."[6]

Steinem's words encapsulate the challenge AIDS poses for feminists. Should we, like her, join the predominantly anti-sex reaction? It is an understandable reaction. Sex has never been completely "safe" for women. When gutter press journalists like Simon Kinnersley try to terrorize and shock *Women's Own* readers ("No one told her that sleeping with a man could be like facing a firing squad . . . no one said that sex could kill . . ."[7]), they convey a message feminists have been hearing for some years from a small but vocal minority in their midst. Sex with men is always and inevitably dangerous, the root cause of men's power over women: "A woman needs a man like a fish needs a harpoon," they might say today.

But for feminists to join the chorus dismissing "the permissive sixties" is for us to betray much that was most radical and important in the sexual politics of women's liberation and wider changes in women's sexual behaviour. It is also to abandon rather than create a sexual climate and practice which could most effectively contain AIDS. It is finally to endorse a reaction which is, in essence, against women's autonomy just as firmly as it is anti-gay and the proponent of a new confining "family" morality. Women's liberation was once well aware that it was women who have always suffered more than men from sexual repression, and the hypocrisy that inevitably accompanies it. Feminists have also always known that, far from being a protection for women, the traditional nuclear family has been a place where the prevalence of child abuse, domestic violence and rape is systematically hidden and denied. Violence within conventional, male-dominated families, as Mary McIntosh succinctly suggests, "is not an extraneous blemish on the social fabric, but part of its warp and weft."[8] The decline of traditional family life and the resulting panic surrounding it comes not so much from the fact that it has been undermined from without by feminism and sexual liberation. It has been undermined from within in response to other social trends. Women with any economic independence– however precarious — are now in a slightly better position to choose to leave unhappy or brutal marriages. The real threat to traditional family life is women's increasing economic independence. (Divorce statistics reveal that 70 per cent of divorces are filed by women and the greater a wife's earnings the more likely a family will break up.[9])

Sexual Politics Then and Now

Historically, women's liberation grew out of the so-called "sexual revolution" of the sixties. The sixties had been a time of increasing public acceptance of sexual relationships and encounters outside marriage. The shift in attitudes resulted from wider social changes which also brought about legal reforms providing easier access to contraception and abortion, facilitating divorce, and partially decriminalizing homosexual relations. Since men have always been sexually active outside marriage, it was most significantly the sexuality of *women* and gay men which was no longer so rigorously policed and punished. The spectre of death or disease from back-street abortion, of shame and dire social penalties for the "fallen woman" who conceived when single — both common in the fifties — no longer haunted the sexual encounters of unmarried but sexually active women. The lowering of sexual restraints did not, as is often suggested, *create* double standards and the blatant sexist objectification of women. It simply *revealed* them as intrinsic to existing sexual mores. That revelation paved the way for the women's liberation movement at the close of the sixties (which, like the contemporary gay liberation movement, was also influenced by the sixties civil rights and student movements).

As I have argued elsewhere,[10] women's liberation in its early days both affirmed and challenged many of the sexual beliefs and practices of the sixties. In affirmation, feminists wanted to explore and express the whole *variety* of their sexual feelings and desires. We wanted to assert an "autonomous" sexuality— free from the customary pressures and coercion from men. In defiance, hetero-sexual feminists challenged sexual practices centred solely on the penis and its performance. And we challenged notions of "masculinity" synonymous with male sexual "conquest" of women. Above all, feminists attacked the ubiquitous language and icono-graphy of sex in our culture, which assigns activity and control to men, passivity and surrender to women.

The existence of so many men's habitual sexual aggression and coercion, however, soon began to overwhelm and undermine this early feminist affirmation of the importance of women's engagement in a joint sexual politics with men. I don't want here to rehearse the bitter splits over sexuality which tore the women's movement apart in the late seventies. I want instead to draw out the relevant implications, from the hopes and heartaches of that earlier time, for a progressive sexual politics today: a politics that can help us understand and surmount the frightening fantasies and restraining realities surrounding AIDS.

First, feminists in the early seventies challenged the "naturalness" of common sense understandings of sexual behaviour. Sex is precisely *not* a simple expression of our animal natures, with men programmed to seek as much sex as possible and women, their passive receptacles, programmed to reproduce. Women too have active sexual desires, and though their outlets may be different from men's, they are no less obsessed by and engaged with the sexual. The huge appeal of romantic literature to women, for example, suggests a steady interest in sexual titillation. Women's sexuality is everywhere more controlled and confined than men's, policed by the legitimation of male sexual coercion in response to any signs of active sexuality in women. But there are no compelling reasons, as women's liberationists once knew (though many feminists today reject this) for seeing women as freer from sexual desire than men. In uncovering and emphasizing the complexity of women's sexual feelings, and the mythology behind assumptions of men's overriding sexual drive, many feminists began to emphasize that sexual behaviour is not simply personal and private but rather historically and socially constructed through public discourses and institutional practices.

Secondly, this earlier sexual politics endorsed and made visible lesbian sexuality. This was the emblem, as it were, of women's autonomous sexuality outside men's control—women's right to choose who and what would turn us on sexually.[11] Heartaches came from the fact that we were less aware at first of how deeply irrational and unconscious forces, going back to childhood, were knotted into out individual histories of sexual longing and ways of relating. Though we might wish to choose who and what would turn us on sexually, those deeper dreams and fantasies proved more durable. The attempt to short circuit this problem at times created its own prescriptive and moralistic dimensions to feminist sexual politics. These problems led some feminists to abandon altogether the search for a new sexual politics. But the complexities of this lived experience could, if approached less voluntaristically, strengthen the feminist commitment to the importance of insisting upon women's rights to explore, understand and express the contradictions of their sexuality. Indeed it seems more important than ever today, in the face of the wider social pressure towards a compulsive and often coercive monogamous heterosexuality.

The third and final aspect of that early sexual politics which remains crucial for us today is the insistence that *men's* behaviour must change. Men who lived with feminists were expected to, and sometimes did, take responsibility for maintaining caring and equal sexual and personal relationships with women, and caring relationships with children. Once again, it was not easy. In particular, men's greater involvement in the home, when it happened, did not undermine their usually greater power and privilege in the world outside. Beyond sexual politics, there were other battles to fight and win: battles which cast a long shadow on domestic and sexual relationships between women and men. But only a minority of feminists then would dismiss the importance of the battle on the home front.

Feminist Responses to AIDS

The crisis surrounding AIDS makes it clear that today we have to push further with those ideas that feminists developed out of the "sexual revolution". Most publicity around AIDS defines sex simply in terms of penetration— for women always the most hazardous, and not necessarily the most rewarding part of it. On every other billboard during the government campaign, as on nearly every TV AIDS "special", sex is once again reduced to the activity of the penis. A penis now newly attired in colourful plastic. It is, as Bea Campbell spelled out, "penetration propaganda", protecting rather than challenging men's historical sexual prerogatives.[12] The "thrust" of the publicity is less sex and fewer partners. Instead, we should be talking about expanding people's notions of sexual relationships and about sexual practices (possible and pleasurable) in situations where we are uncertain whether we or our partners are free from contact with HIV.

It is intensely depressing that even apparently liberal approaches to AIDS education today — like ITV's *First AIDS* programme for young people — still endorse rather than question the most macho and heterosexist conceptions of sexuality. The aim of *First AIDS* was solely to force young men to use condoms, enlisting the support of young women. The experts all endorsed the idea that young men were driven to fuck, the more often the better. They sat back while the presenter ignored or mocked the few young men who were ready to explore the differences between macho mythologies and their own experience.

Yet surely AIDS gives us reason and space to re-think the primitive but powerful symbol of the male sexual beast, the myth so central to maintaining existing ideologies and practices of male domination? Any more serious study of sexual fantasy and behaviour would uncover something very different from this mythology. It would uncover endless complexity: the interplay of an amazing variety of physical contacts and emotional needs and desires in both women and men, needs and desires combining the longings, fears, humiliations, self-love and self-loathing we have experienced or imagined in our intimate contacts with others throughout a lifetime. As every feminist once shouted from the roof tops, sex is not simply penis-in-vagina penetration. Even sex researchers in their limited, mechanistic way, have revealed that women orgasm more readily with clitoral stimulation, while sex therapists find it useful to outlaw penetration at certain times and encourage the exploration of other sensual pleasures instead. There are no intrinsic boundaries to sexual pleasure. Sex is every conceivable intimate pleasure our heads can dream up. It is the mind which is the dominant sex organ.

The overwhelming problem in facing the challenge of AIDS is the continuing *significance*, not the *decline*, of guilt and secrecy about sex. It is the fact that it is still hard for us to talk openly and honestly about sex. This, in turn, is the product of other continuities in thought and practices surrounding sex. It connects with the continuing reality of men's power over women: how this is manifested, symbolized and strengthened in the language and practice of sex. Men fear what they see as "feminine" in themselves (which includes talking about feelings and relationships); women deny and repress their own interest in sex. Yet men as well as women would benefit from becoming more emotionally articulate (silence is no longer sexy). It might even lower the compulsion and fear of failure which accompanies men's sexuality. It would certainly lower the danger that accompanies women's sexuality, and begin to relieve the most basic frustration of making it with men: communicatio interrupta.

AIDS also makes lethal nonsense of the attempts by the moral right to end sex education in schools. We should be pushing for imaginative sex education in all schools, fostering the fullest possible discussion around all aspects of sex from primary school onwards. Along with realizing that it is not distinctive *types* of people who are at risk from AIDS, we need to think about the fluidity of sexual categories generally. The differences in types of people with respect to AIDS is not in their sexual preferences or practices as such, but rather in whether they take responsibility for the risks others might face in sexual encounters or relationships with them.

There is a lot we can learn from the organized gay reaction to the AIDS epidemic in the West. In San Francisco it is estimated that 95 per cent of gay men now follow safe sex practices. Fewer gay men than heterosexual men there are now contracting sexually transmitted diseases and the incidence of new people becoming HIV positive is dropping rapidly (*Economist*, 23 August 1986). The Terrence Higgins Trust here, following the success of gay advice work in the US, has always advocated a positive and open attitude towards sex: "SEX IS GOOD, IT'S FUN, IT'S UP TO ALL OF US NOT TO SPOIL IT . . . be inventive sexually . . . get into wanking, massage and fantasies. There's more to sex than just fucking . . . make sure your partner wears a condom [if] you want to fuck . . ." David Rampton wrote a short account in the *Mail on Sunday* in 1986 describing how AIDS has changed his attitudes to sex as a happily single gay men: "I found myself looking at what I was doing, asking if I was liking it, and finding out how I could continue to enjoy it without taking any risks . . . Then came the memorable occasion when I spent the night with somebody, and I suddenly realized I hadn't had to consciously think about keeping to what is safe. And that was a real breakthrough, because it meant that I'd become comfortable with safe sex and enjoyed the positive, imaginative side of it, rather than just being stuck with the negative, difficult side of it all."

Sadly the Trust's advice booklet, written by women for women, does not take a similarly clear pro-sex stance. It in no way counters the prevailing idea that women are inherently less interested in sex than men. It is as though women's sexual role today — rather like the agenda for the Victorian lady — is to help control men's sexuality and avoid catching diseases. Surely, now more than ever, women need to combat the misleading image and rhetoric of "testosterone man" with more positive, woman-centred ideas of sexuality. In graphic and witty contrast *Making It: A Woman's Guide to Sex in the Age of AIDS* by US AIDS activists Cindy Patton and Janis Kelly is positive and pro-sex throughout.[13] They describe some of the AIDS educational activities groups of women in the US have begun, pointing out that learning to feel good about safer sex and sorting out problems with partners is often easier with a bit of help from your friends. Educational activities include, for example, the ranking exercise: "Give each woman a card with a way of having sex on it (be explicit). Everyone then lines up in a row from 'most safe' to 'most dangerous' activity . . . this exercise will help you learn to think out what is safe and what is not, and how to talk about risk."[14] Of course, in ways that are anathema to all the usual penetrative and anti-sex propaganda, it might also give you many new ideas on what is safe and sexy.

Penetrative sex is riskier for heterosexual women than men. Men pass HIV to women or men more easily than women can pass it to men. (The body fluids containing the T4 cells which carry HIV are mainly concentrated in semen and blood, vaginal and cervical secretions contain fewer of these cells.) This does not mean that women who enjoy it should abandon vaginal or anal sex — nor more casual sexual encounters. It does mean that women should avoid men (or women) who take no responsibility for their partners in sex. We cannot all propel ourselves into trusted monogamous relationships, even if we may want to. And to advise young women to wait for "Mr Right" (who just might be HIV positive anyway), in line with government propaganda, is to encourage their subordination, passivity and repression or denial of their sexuality. It is to increase their vulnerability and uncertainties with men. In contrast, encouraging young women to explore their own sexuality may well decrease their willingness to agree to certain types of sexual encounters which give little pleasure. (Women who are unsure of their male partners should also use the spermicide Nonoxynol 9, present in most contraceptive foams, which kills the human immunodeficiency virus on contact.)

There have so far in Britain been few or no cases of lesbian HIV transmission. But it is very misleading to suggest, as does the lesbian separatist journal *Gossip*, that AIDS is only "marginally a lesbian issue". Lesbians clearly face similar risks to heterosexual women via partners who may have directly or indirectly picked up the virus through intravenous drug taking or via bisexual women or lesbians working as prostitutes. (The US Women's AIDS Network recommends that lesbians at risk use latex barriers [squares of thin rubber] for oral sex and finger cots [sheaths for the fingers] for hand to genital contact.)[15]

A feminist sexual politics and the challenge of AIDS require a sexual climate as imaginative, as egalitarian, as guilt-free and as knowledgeable as possible. However, what we are confronting is government and media campaigns fostering a generalized anxiety about sex.[16] We also face a callous and brutal disregard for the needs of those already HIV positive, a vicious blaming and persecution of people with AIDS (regally endorsed by Princess Anne), which can serve only to stifle rational thought and action on the best way of containing the virus. A more appropriate and effective response would be to insist that this government make any discrimination against those who are HIV positive illegal, whether in jobs, housing or insurance, thus giving them prompt access to advice, assistance and treatment when they need it. As important is combating a climate of guilt and fear where people are more likely to be paralysed by the threat of AIDS than propelled into sensible action. This government could act as energetically to counter the current homophobic and "victim"-blaming reaction in the tabloid press as it has to publicize the dangers of AIDS. In fact, of course, it is doing the reverse: Section 28 of the Local Government Act is an attempt to sanction official manifestations of homophobia.

An internationalist perspective is also essential for facing the challenge of AIDS. Rather than imagining, for example, that heterosexual transmission of AIDS will be mainly confined to Africa — and can be dismissed with a few racist jokes about African sexual practices — we need to insist that our government puts pressure on the EEC to invest massively in health care in Africa. The catastrophic spread of AIDS in that continent, where few black nations can afford even to screen the blood used in transfusions for the virus, creates an international health risk.

Any successful campaign against AIDS, which will have to come from all of us and not just from governments, will be one which re-educates everyone, women and men alike, but particularly men, to combine sexual activity with responsibility and concern for others. Fear in itself never did stop sexually transmitted diseases from spreading, as the history of syphilis should warn us. Some people find danger — even the threat of death — a sexual turn-on. Others, however, suffer so much crippling anxiety around sex that doctors are seriously worried about the spread of AIDS *phobia*, with increasing numbers of patients who cannot be reassured even when declared AIDS-free.

Perhaps the biggest question we face today is how heterosexual men, who have yet to be politicized as a sexual community, can be educated to behave responsibly towards women as sexual partners. Health authorities in the US are officially concerned that hetero-sexual men will not so readily care for others and — more importantly — be educated with the same ease as homosexuals, since there is not the same network of friendships and com-munication.[17] "Can you trust the boys?" asked AIDS information officer David Panter in youth clubs and schools in the inner London borough of Islington in 1987. "No," was the deafening reply, from an audience where girls sat in rapt attention while the boys became embarrassed and giggled, or drifted away.[18] The whole context of women's and men's heterosexual encounters and relationships will need to change to meet the challenge of AIDS.

Some women — younger women particularly — and perhaps a few men are beginning to realize this. AIDS could serve as a spur, not for more of the same evasion and hypocrisy around sex, but for more equal sexual relations between women and men and the recognition of sexual diversity. This will not take us back to any coercive heterosexual family morality — not once both women and men are able to discuss with honesty their sexual preferences and practices. A sexual politics and climate which promotes "good sex", in this sense, is more likely to produce "safe sex" than any reassertion of a morally conservative politics of denial, guilt and fear.

Will the boys start listening once the girls start leaving those who don't? Will straight men learn from the sexual politics and practices of an already politicized gay community? Maybe they will have to. And then the sexual revolution can begin in earnest. Fighting for women's autonomy and power and combating homophobia is part of the same international "conspiracy" of sexual radicals. The right has always known it. It's time for feminists and the left to catch up with them. It is also, as it happens, the most effective way to meet the challenge of AIDS.

Notes

1. Frances Fitzgerald, *Cities on a Hill*, London 1987 p. 12.

2. Graham Hancock, "Why AIDS Matters", *The New Internationalist*, no. 169, March 1987, p. 5.

3. See *Panos Document*, no. 1, London 1986.

4. For exceptions see Susan Ardill, "AIDS", *Spare Rib*, January 1987; Sue O'Sullivan, "What Do You Think about AIDS?", *Spare Rib*, February 1987; Lesley Dike, "AIDS: What Women Should Know", *Outwrite*, no. 54, January 1987.

5. Erica Jong, "Is all the Hysteria a Blessing in Disguise?", *Good Housekeeping*, November 1986, p. 65.

6. Quoted in Katherine Whitehorn, "How AIDS is Changing Women's Lives", *The Observer*, 22 February 1988, p.53.

7. Simon Kinnersley, "You Don't Need to be a Drug Addict, a Homosexual or a Prostitute . . . to Catch AIDS", *Women's Own*, July 12 1986, p. 18.

8. Mary McIntosh, "Family Secrets: Child Sexual Abuse", *The Chartist*, January 1988.

9. See Andrew Hacker, "Farewell to the Family?" *New York Review of Books*, vol. xxlx, no. 10, 18 March 1982, pp. 37–45; and Andrew Cherlin, *Marriage Divorce Remarriage*, Harvard 1982.

10. Lynne Segal, *Is the Future Female* ?, London 1987, esp. ch. 3.

11. See for example Bea Campbell, "Sexuality and Submission", *Red Rag*, no. 5, 1973.

12. Bea Campbell, "Bealine", *Marxism Today*, December 1987, p. 9.

13. Cindy Patton and Janis Kelly *Making It: A Woman's Guide to Sex in the Age of AIDS*, New York 1987.

14. Ibid, p. 16.

15. Lesley Dike, "AIDS: What Women Should Know", *Outwrite*, no. 54, January 1987, p. 10.

16. Simon Watney, *Policing Desire: Pornography, AIDS and the Media*, London 1987.

17. See *The Economist*, August 1986, p. 33.

18. Quoted in Ben Burrell and Fiona Murray, "Young Love and the AIDS Factor", *The Guardian*, March 1987.

JAN ZITA GROVER

CONSTITUTIONAL SYMPTOMS

I was trained as an historian. I bring what that discipline taught me to my personal and professional life within and around AIDS. For the past two years, I have worked as a fly on the wall of the establishment, as a medical editor on an AIDS textbook project at San Francisco General Hospital. During that time, I have also worked as a volunteer for the Shanti Project (San Francisco) and the AIDS Project of the East Bay (Alameda County). Among long-time personal friends and friends I have made on these projects, I have listened to men talk about their anticipated deaths, seen their deaths, watched people await their HIV antibody test results, seen the fallout in my own and friends' lives when we have taken too much on ourselves or when we have chastized ourselves for taking on too little. I've attended conferences —medical, political, cultural, left, right — on AIDS. I have lectured and written about AIDS, explaining time and again to myself and others how this epidemic is different from and similar to others, and why as a lesbian and feminist I am involved in it.

I mention all this in order to situate myself somewhat in relation to what follows: two fragments of what I fear will be a lifelong project of trying to understand how AIDS fits into pre-existing categories in our lives and how it has expanded, exploded, vanquished other cultural categories. The first, "Incontinent Nostalgia", is a note on something I've noticed only in the past year: evidences of growing nostalgia/fantasy about "the old days" of AIDS, when individuals, not institutions, seemed at the centre of community response. The second note, "The Necessity of Metaphor", addresses the impossibility of conceiving AIDS *except* through the category of metaphor. Unlike Susan Sontag's injunction that we strip disease of its (disabling) metaphors, I argue that disease is *only* knowable through its metaphors. And while it therefore behoves us to select and reject those on offer very carefully, we can only understand what is largely invisible, intangible, through the function of language and imagery.

Neither of these notes draws any conclusions. Instead, these are notes toward what I hope is my eventual coming-to-terms with AIDS in those future days when its survivors will constitute a generation-within-a-generation — a cohort in lifelong mourning and wonderment over what we have passed through.

Incontinent Nostalgia

If there is one thing certain about "the organic community," it is that it has always gone.

Raymond Williams, *Culture and Society* [1]

In *Awakenings,* Oliver Sacks describes encephalitic persons whose virus-induced slumbers — some of them thirty or forty years in length — were disturbed in the mid 1960s by the administration of L-DOPA, the precursor of the nerve-transmitter dopamine. The physiological and emotional *awakening* [2] prompted by this drug caused several encephalitic people to suffer an overwhelming grief for the past — for the only fully meaningful, historical present in which they had even dwelt: a long-gone present in which they had experienced love, sex, fashion, friendship. So painful was the contrast between the impoverished world into which one patient, Rosa R., had been reborn — "a time gap beyond comprehension or bearing," Sacks calls it — that she begged to be returned to her encephalitic "sleep". Sacks termed Rosa R.'s inability to leave behind her vivid youth for her impoverished present "incontinent nostalgia".

I want to talk here about another condition we might term incontinent nostalgia, this having to do with AIDS. I am not speaking of the understandable nostalgia for that past which predates AIDS — a period in which sex for most people had fewer and less mortal consequences, a period in which gay culture opened and expanded, in which fine young men and women were not dying by the hundreds, infants and mothers were not mortally infected and parents were rarely burying their children. These are important reasons for regret, ones that are being documented movingly from within grieving communities in fiction, video, and film — most particularly from within gay male communities. The incontinent nostalgia I want to address here is something else — that of individuals who did early work with people with AIDS and now find themselves either burned out, turned out, or turned off — sometimes all three —by the evolution of AIDS service into professional organizations, into what increasingly is being termed the "AIDS establishment".

In saying this, I recognize and indeed wish to emphasize that the occasions for my observations also mean a great many other things, depending upon who is doing the viewing and to what ends. But the AIDS epidemic is, unfortunately, now old enough that it is generating its own social history, and this is fixed not so much upon that never-never land that predates AIDS (as it was even two years ago) as it is upon the earliest days of the epidemic.[3]

The evidence of this phenomenon is everywhere. Cindy Patton's paper "The AIDS Industry"[4] is an attack on the AIDS establishment and what she perceives as the incursion of middle-class hetero-sexual men and women into organizations that had originally been supported and staffed by lesbians and gay men.[4] Patton's measure of the distance travelled from the past was the disappearance of the small, hardy band of grassroots activists — the organic community of like-minded persons caring for their own.

In April 1988, the San Francisco Human Rights Commission filed a formal complaint against the Shanti Project, the city's largest AIDS service organization, for possible discrimination against women and ethnic minorities. The fact that such charges are now pending against Shanti points to several things: the bitterness of ex-employees at finding in Shanti not an organic community but a hierarchical organization; the differing commitment of more recent employees, who view the project more as an employer and a possible route or obstacle to a career than as a cause; the perceived isolation and solidification of power/authority in a core of old-timers; the resistance of a (gay, white) establishment to challenges and demand for participation on the part of women, Latinos, blacks, and other, more recent AIDS "constituencies".

The disaffections beginning to be voiced in our communities about the large service organizations are necessary. Their implicit model is that of the for-profit capitalist corporation with its vast disparity in income and power between officers and a majority of employees, its emphasis upon models of efficiency and productivity drawn, again, from profit-making industry via government funding agencies, its conviction that it can be all things to all people if it just does a little judicious minority hiring and outreach.[6]

Moreover, there is little question that the appropriation of both "volunteer" discourse and funding by the large (and largely gay, white, middle-class) AIDS groups makes it more difficult for smaller, newer and, most particularly, minority groups to get attention, authority, and money for their work.

What I am drawing attention to here is something different, however: the uses of the past (the past that never was) in criticizing, justifying, rationalizing the present — what Williams termed: "An idealization, based on a temporary situation and a deep desire for stability, served to cover and to evade the actual and bitter contradictions of the time."[7]

The uses of the past must rationalize and smooth over the "contradictions" of both the present and the past. Thus the early days of AIDS organizing and care must be made to appear more heroic, more fraught with crisis, but withall more closely-knit and unified, than the present, with its divisive politics.[8]

Other examples of the past-made-perfect come to mind. Media attention focused on Peter Duesberg's conservative model for AIDS can be read in part as a yearning for the simplicities of disease-models past and the reassurances of conspiracy theory. The New York *Native* and other gay papers have paid considerable adulatory attention to Duesberg, the UC-Berkeley molecular biologist who believes that HIV (human immunodeficiency virus) is not the aetiological agent of AIDS. Their fascination with Duesberg seems based not so much on his argument, which is tenuous and unsubstantiated,[9] as on his position as an outsider to the AIDS establishment — that is, to centres of endowed research like the National Institutes of Health, New York City's Memorial Sloane Kettering Institute, San Francisco General Hospital, and their researchers — whom he enjoys goading for their self-interest and careerism.[10] "Where are the days when the only people researching AIDS were our friends?" the gay Duesberg partisans seem to cry.[11]

It is a measure of the hostility aroused in gay circles by the medical/research world of placebo-controlled trials, tail-dragging FDA approval of investigational new-drug protocols, and ambitious young physicians making their mark in AIDS, that these same gay activists ignore Duesberg's own (homophobic) speculation that AIDS is the result of an immune exhaustion brought on by irresponsible living. But as one of the first scientists to voice the scepticism so widely felt in gay AIDS circles, Duesberg does have an audience.

But it is a soft, unexamined fall-back: Duesberg and the "syphilis connection" theorists offer only the comforts and seductions of the already-known: Koch's postulates applied to life-forms undreamt of in Koch's day and infections/treatments regarded as safely familiar and therefore manageable, controllable.

And what of the claims that AIDS has become an industry, that it is severed from its grassroots origins in radical gay politics? Like the seduction of the syphilis connection, such arguments seem founded on an ahistoric reading of the present — on an insistence that the shape of the present resemble the shape of the past. Groups like ACT UP, ACT NOW and ADAPT are the crisis-seven-years-later analogues of the informal safer-sex educators and buddy-systems of 1982–1983, parented equally by grassroots organizations and the large service organizations they are meant to challenge or complement. And are all AIDS researchers with government contracts or university affiliations sell-outs to the US government's (passively) genocidal AIDS policies, the federal Food and Drug Administration and National Institute of Health's infighting? Here again, the answer is no — many are actively complicit, some actively participate in underground drug supplies, compassionate AIDS diagnoses for people with debilitating symptoms of HIV infection. Is everyone working for a mainstream AIDS organization — Shanti in San Francisco, AIDS Project of Los Angeles, Gay Men's Health Crisis in New York City, Terrence Higgins Trust in London — an unwitting dupe of the AIDS industry or a crypto-conservative doing his or her jolly Reaganite/Thatcherite private-charity thing? Or can we not imagine instead the messy, even contradictory reality: that many of these "official" volunteers are also members of ACT UP, members of the grey- and black-market drug trade, or unofficial AIDS service organizations.

We run a great risk in characterizing people's identities and motivations in order to comfort ourselves, to impose order on confusion. If as gay men, lesbians, feminists, we have learned with great pain to reject the notion of an essential, integrated self — the pain of losing social/sexual/political continuity and acceptance in our larger communities, then we should extend no cruder readings to the commitment of others fighting AIDS. These too are multiple, contradictory, expedient, fractured. The scepticism we bring to our readings of mainstream history-making must extend to our own projective fantasies of golden ages, organic communities, dissident scientists, magic bullets.

The Necessity of Metaphor

My point is that illness is not a metaphor, and that the most truthful way of regarding illness - and the healthiest way of being ill — is one most purified of, most resistant to, metaphoric thinking.

Susan Sontag, *Illness As Metaphor* [12]

This is Susan Sontag's starting-point in her examination of the language used to describe cancer. It is a starting-point itself constructed as an extended metaphor:

Illness is the night-side of life, a more onerous citizenship. Everyone who is born holds dual citizenship, in the kingdom of the well and in the kingdom of the sick. Although we all prefer to use only the good passport, sooner or later each of us is obliged, at least for a spell, to identify ourselves as citizens of that other place.[14]

I point this out not as an indication of Sontag's inconsistency in applying her own standards, but as a measure of the impossibility of what she calls for: the eradication of metaphor as a medium of understanding.

But language is itself metaphor, and we can no more "purify" it in discussing disease than in describing a beautiful day or how love makes us feel. Constructing less devastating ways of "regarding illness" is not simply a matter of promoting ideas of sickness "resistant to . . . metaphoric thinking." Rather, it is assessing what's available metaphorically, what the implications of current metaphors may be for various audiences, and who benefits from those conceits most commonly at work in media, medicine, politics, and public health.

As Sontag has pointed out,[15] cancer has been popularly and medically metaphorized as a *war*, replete with battles, skirmishes, victims, and heroes.[16] The usefulness of this metaphor in describing the unknown may account for its common usage; we have not only war on cancer, but wars on drugs, wars on crime, wars on juvenile delinquency, wars on poverty, wars on hypertension, wars on sickle-cell anemia, wars on mental illness. So commonplace, in fact, is the conceit of war in discussions/actions on issues of public concern that its *absence* in the case of AIDS becomes a particularly signifying absence or silence.

What does it mean *not* to have AIDS constructed in terms of "a war against . . ."? What metaphors have been used instead, and what are the significances of their use?

We might first consider how the dominant medical metaphor, "a war against . . .", functions as it is commonly used in public discourse. In the examples above, for one thing, we (we-who-are-addressed as well as we-who-do-the-speaking/acting) are all (presumably) allied against that-which-is-warred-upon: there is a common alliance (us) against a common if wholly abstracted enemy (poverty, cancer, etc.). Sacrifice is expected; failure is expected (hence victims, heroes), but the enemy's hostages or victims — the poor, the diseased — will eventually be won over to our side, become one with us. And what of those who fall in battle? That's the price of winning, the price of glory.

War as a metaphoric construction for social relations allows users and audience access to a rich vocabulary of secondary signifiers drawn from historical wars: the Trojan Horse, pyrrhic victory, crossing the Rubicon, the Holocaust, the second (or third) front, colonial wars, tactics, strategies. These, in turn, make more tangible the abstract processes of scientific theory, biological research, medical treatment, and subjective feeling.[17] Pitched at the level of popular public discourse, the historical resonances invoked by war metaphors prove self-fulfilling: with drugs, we may "win the battle but lose the war," with cancer we may "kill the messenger who brings the bad news" (e.g. the surgeon general's warnings on cancer-and-smoking, cholesterol-and-heart disease) or explain the devastations of chemotherapy by recurring to one of the absurdist horrors of the Viet Nam war — "destroying the [patient] in order to save him." Metaphors normalize the unfamiliar, domesticate it. In the case of processes widely anathematized (terminal illness, drug addiction), metaphors provide rationale and precedent for invasion, occupation, and normalization of *the enemy* — the diseased body, the diseased "personality".

The prevailing metaphors for AIDS are not of war: they are contamination — sexual contamination. Alain Corbin has described how prostitution in nineteenth-century France was discussed, in fiction, medicine, religion, legislation, and public-health edicts, largely in terms of "pre-Pasteurian mythologies" of putrefaction and sewerage.[18] This was an enabling metaphor: by embracing it, those who told it and those who listened to it acknowledged the need for containing the contamination. Such a metaphor is not as abstracting as that of war — contamination always presumes a personalized source — nor does it assume an eventual winning-over to our side. That is not its goal: the goal is to keep the other side as far away from us as possible, to keep it as unlike us as possible. The metaphor of contamination does not suppose the normalization of the source of infection: it supposes only its containment, for contamination is not so much anthropomorphic (as the enemy is) as it is anti-human, even anti-natural.

Nature, it turns out, is the last refuge of the scoundrel: a lesson taught profoundly and variously by Jeffrey Weeks and Michel Foucault[19] in connection with sexual practices, sexual identities, and with AIDS expanded to include other sources of social unease. When all else fails the mainstream commentator on AIDS, s/he still has at disposal the seemingly irrefutable argument that x or y is unnatural and therefore deserves or inevitably brings on Nature's revenge for (name your vice): promiscuity, homosexuality, non-reproductive (usually anal) sex, drug-use.[20] It is this category of the unnatural that gives the shape to the threat of contamination, of spread and leakage.

Arguments based upon epidemiological evidence have little effect upon popular/media constructions of the epidemic that are grounded in belief in the unnatural origin and growth of AIDS. In the worlds imagined by social and political conservatives, AIDS is more akin in its imagery and implications to *Invasion of the Body Snatchers* and its new life forms than to previous earthly epidemics. In this language-world, HIV becomes either impossibly difficult or disarmingly easy to contract — depending on who you are. For like evangelical protestantism, AIDS appears as something one is either saved from or not, less a result of specific practices enacted or avoided than a state of the individual's naturalness/grace or unnaturalness/sin.[21]

Evidences of this construction of AIDS abound not only in written texts but in the visual discourse on AIDS.[22] What, we might ask, constitutes a meaningful photograph of a person with AIDS? Is it a portrait of that person before physical signs and symptoms mark him/her (but what of the latent infection)? A portrait of that person with the physical signs and symptoms of illness or chemotherapy (but what of the person who looks healthy to the end)? A portrait of that person in extremis? All of these? None of these?

The choices made by mainstream media favour the protestant either-or, grace-or-sin sketched above. I readily concede that identity of any sort is inherently unstable and that still photography is a resistant medium for exploring this fact. But the photographic coverage of AIDS by for instance *Newsweek, Time, US News & World Report*, as well as by daily newspapers, has made little attempt to reflect the instability of human identity vis à vis AIDS. *Newsweek's* "The Faces of AIDS" issue (10 August 1987), for example, mixes snapshots of people who died of AIDS that were taken before, during, and at the end of their lives. This appears to have been a tactical necessity if the essay was to include depictions of these people at all. But the peculiar effect of these twelve pages of head-shots and high-school yearbook-like descriptions ("Patrick Dillree, 26. Hairdresser, Minneapolis. He believed he got AIDS from his IV cocaine habit; Anthony Izewski, 34. Property management, Los Angeles. 'Tony enriched the lives of those around him'; Nina Johnson, 77. Wilmington, Del. A transfusion case whom nurses refused to touch.") is to make these people look as if they didn't know what hit them (failed grace) or to make their appearance a consequence of the moral failings often attributed to them (wages of sin). In the format of the police mug-shot or the yearbook, the causes and consequences of AIDS are contained.

Extended photojournalist essays on people with AIDS make the problems of the dominant contamination-containment metaphor even clearer. Conventionally, a young man is shown, presumably pre-HIV infection, in a snapshot or formal portrait — smiling, radiant with the markers of health. We then follow his days as "a victim" with all the markers of sickness — hospital visits, hospital rooms,

garbed attendants, wasted body, possibly other bodily markers of
AIDS — Kaposi's sarcoma, lymphatic shunting, loss of hair. The risks
that underlie his downcast state are presented not as viral but moral
in origin — drug addiction, homosexuality. The implication is that
those of us who are resistant to these or other "vices" (coded as
risks) are also resistant to AIDS.[23] At the same time, we have a right to
be alarmed at the presence or incursion of the contaminated in our
midst.[24] If this all sounds very familiar — homosexuality as a moral
taint but at the same time as something contagious and therefore
containable — we come to the heart of the dominant metaphorizing
around AIDS: its unnatural nature.

Notes

1. Raymond Williams, *Culture and Society: 1780–1950*, London 1958, p. 159. By
tracing the idea of rustic "organic communities" backward in time, Williams
movingly and convincingly demystified the ahistoric impulse to locate longed-for
cultural values and practices in the past. The full exposition of this project appears in
his later *The Country and the City*, London 1973.

2. Oliver Sacks, *Awakenings*, New York 1983. Sacks employs the term awakenings
because the chemotherapy and music therapy he describes "recall Parkinsonians
from inactivity (or abnormal activity) into normal activity, and from the abyss of
unbeing into normal being. 'Qui non agit non existit,' when the Parkisonian is not
active he does not exist — when we recall him to activity we recall him to life," (p.
292, fn. 1).

3. An interesting case in point is the published short fiction on AIDS by British and
US gay male writers which has appeared in two recent collections: George
Stambolian, ed., *Men on Men*, New York 1986, and Edmund White and Adam
Mars-Jones, *The Darker Proof: Stories from a crisis*, New York 1988. Particularly in the
latter collection, there is a noticeable tendency in White to focus upon a nostalgia for
life before AIDS and in Mars-Jones to a resolute immersion in life after AIDS. It is
possible, of course, that these emphases may be an artifact of editorial selection.

4. see this volume, pages 113 to 125.

5. Charles Linebarger, "Job Bias Alleged at Shanti Project", San Francisco *Sentinel*, 8
April 1988, pp. 1, 12.

6. A long-overdue analysis of this uncritical use of the for-profit corporation as a
model for government and public-good agencies is Robert Lekachman, *Visions and
Nightmares: America after Reagan*, New York 1987. Lekachman's argument is
excerpted in "The craze for privatization: dubious social results of a Reaganite
dogma," *Dissent*, summer 1987, pp. 302–7.

7. Williams, *The Country and the City*, p. 45.

8. Randy Shilts *And the Band Played On*, New York 1987, plays this theme up to the

hilt. See Rose Applebaum, "AIDS exposé paints vivid picture — but watch out for what's missing," *Frontline*, 15 February 1988, pp. 6–7, for an excellent review of the history Shilts left out of his account of AIDS, 1981–1985.

9. See for instance, William Booth, "A Rebel Without a Cause of AIDS," *Science*, 25 March 1988, pp. 1485–8, for the only careful discussion of Duesberg's claims and AIDS HIV researchers counter-claims to appear in the journal-world in which Duesberg first argued against HIV. Through the science-journal grapevine, I understand that individual AIDS researchers are preparing refutations.

10. See Ann Guidici Fettner's piece on Duesberg, "Dealing with Duesberg: bad science makes strange bedfellows," *Village Voice*, 2 February 1988, and Booth, op. cit.

11. In pro-Duesberg articles, Duesberg is invariably described in resonantly left-progressive terms as a "dissident scientist", "outsider", or "gadfly", as if the very terms writers append to him constituted his moral claim (see for example Rex Wockner, "Dissident scientists battle AIDS dogma," *In These Times*, 4 May 1988, p. 5). The *Native*'s and *In These Times*' coverage of Duesberg lays the burden of proof not on his airy challenges but rather on "the AIDS establishment". In popular media coverage, little or no attention is given to the epidemiological studies that have played so large a part in constructing a paradigm for AIDS that includes HIV. Instead, all studies become suspect because "egos", "conspiracies", and "cover-ups" may be involved — except Duesberg's.

12. Susan Sontag, *Illness as Metaphor*, New York 1978, p. 3.

13. Sontag, loc. cit.

14. Cf. Sontag, op. cit., pp. 64–7.

15. Sontag remarks that unlike the warlike imagery describing cancer in the twentieth century, tuberculosis in the nineteenth was metaphorized largely in economic terms: "unregulated, abnormal, incoherent growth . . . TB is described in images that sum up the negative behaviour of nineteenth-century *homo economicus*: consumption; wasting; squandering of vitality" (pp. 62–3).

16. That these two central conceits are drawn from different historical periods is at least as significant as their metaphoric dissimilarity. The fact that Republican presidents' "war on drugs," Democratic "wars on poverty," legislative "wars on illiteracy," etc., are also conceived in bellicose terms — as is the "war/fight against heart disease/hypertension/birth defects" — should suggest that it is war as a human condition that constitutes a twentieth-century structure of feeling. Such a structure can and does fit a variety of social facts to its ideological framework — not just the idea of cancer.

17. Albert Einstein, for example, created visual metaphors to propose and understand; language followed to summarize what he discovered through images. In a letter to Jacques Hadamard [n.d.]: "The words or the language, as they are written or spoken, do not seem to play any role in my mechanism of thought. The psychical entities which seem to serve as elements in thought are certain signs and more or less clear images which can be 'voluntarily' reproduced or combined . . . The above mentioned elements are, in my case, of visual and some of muscular type. Conventional words or other signs have to be sought for laboriously only in a secondary stage, when the mentioned associative play is sufficiently established . . ." Quoted in *The Creative Process*, ed. Brewster Ghiselin, New York 1952, p. 43. See also Albert Einstein, *The World As I see It*, 1935, and *Out of My Later Years*, 1950.

18. Alain Corbin, "Commercial sexuality in nineteenth-century France: a system of

images and regulations," *The Making of the Modern Body: sexuality and society in the nineteenth century* (ed. Catherine Gallagher and Thomas Laqueur), Berkeley 1987, pp. 209–19.

19. For example, Michel Foucault, *The History of Sexuality* and Jeffrey Weeks, *Sexuality and Its Discontents*, both of which describe and analyze the ways in which the categories *Nature* and *the natural* have been used to stigmatize and delimit the boundaries of "acceptable" sexualities.

20. See, variously, Art Ulene, M.D., *Safe Sex in a Dangerous World: Understanding and coping with the threat of AIDS*, New York; Helen Singer Kaplan, M.D., Ph.D., *The Real Truth About Women and AIDS: How to eliminate the risks without giving up love and sex*, New York 1987; William Masters, M.D., Virginia Johnson, and Robert Kolodny, M.D., *Crisis: Heterosexual behaviour in the age of AIDS*, New York 1988; Graham Hancock and Enver Carim, *AIDS: The deadly epidemic*, London 1986. Among US popular weekly periodicals, *Newsweek* has provided the most continuous (and inconsistent) coverage of AIDS; see J. Z. Grover, "*Newsweek* covers AIDS," *Extra!*, New York in press; J. Z. Grover, "The AIDS bureaucracy and other deadly disorders," *In These Times*, 4–10 May 1988, pp. 18–19; J. Z. Grover, "A matter of life and death," *The Women's Review of Books* (March 1988), pp. 1, 3; entire issue of *Radical America*, 20:6, September 1987.

21. One of the fascinating aspects of current popular discourse around *the heterosexual threat* is its mutually-cancelling propositions: on the one hand (e.g., Michael A. Fumento: "AIDS: Are heterosexuals at Risk?" *Commentary*, November 1987, pp. 21–27; Edward M. Brecher, "Straight sex, AIDS, and the mixed-up press", *Columbia Journalism Review*, March–April 1988, pp. 46–50), commentators accuse predominantly gay-male AIDS organizations of exaggerating the threat of the HIV epidemic to heterosexuals in order to garner support for their own needs; on the other (e.g., Helen Singer Kaplan, *The Real Truth About Women and AIDS*), gay men are accused of underplaying the epidemic's threat in order to keep services focused on their own needs at the expense of women and children.

22. Important work on this topic has been done by Simon Watney. See, e.g. *Policing Desire: Pornography, AIDS, and the Media*, London 1987, and "Visual AIDS: advertising ignorance," *New Socialist*, March 1987, reprinted *Radical America* 20:6 (September 1987), pp. 79–82.

23. *Newsweek's The Faces of AIDS* is fascinating in this regard — where a biographical bit was unavailable or otherwise unuseable, editors used the descriptive space beneath each "face" to insert the "risk practice" that presumably precipitated that person's death: e.g., "A bisexual, he was engaged to be married"; "A haemophiliac, he was planning to become a doctor"; "She was infected by her bisexual fiancé"; "An IV-drug user, she had two children"; "He died, as did his mother, from a contaminated blood transfusion"; "A drug addict." It is difficult to read these slogans and not see them as an us versus them, saved versus damned litany.

24. *Newsweek's* latest horror story, "The gay refugees: seeking an AIDS oasis on the great plains" (9 May 1988, pp. 20, 25), provides an anecdotal account of the (unnumbered) gay men "who are seeking refuge from AIDS in the remote reaches of the West." According to the article, filed by John McCormick in North Dakota, gay men are moving to North Dakota, Wyoming, Montana, South Dakota and Idaho. No

figures or other solid evidence are provided for this "lifestyle" piece, which offers a photograph of a gay bar (along with its name) in North Dakota.

This piece does not begin to fulfil responsible journalism in documenting a movement it may well be inventing. Its only verifiable facts are the number of reported cases of AIDS in these states, which bear no substantive relationship to the speculations in the article. What the piece does is sound the familiar media alarm around containment/contamination — "homosexuals are drawn to the Great Plains."

MEURIG HORTON

BUGS, DRUGS AND PLACEBOS

The Opulence of Truth, or how to make a treatment decision in an epidemic

On Sunday, 30 November 1988, a remarkable meeting took place at the Body Positive centre in Earls Court, London. Remarkable because it was a meeting between medical researchers wishing to conduct a drug trial, and prospective trial participants, the subjects of research. Remarkable because it was probably the first such encounter within the annals of British medicine. The seminar was arranged by the Medical Research Council (MRC) working party, Body Positive, and the Terrence Higgins Trust.[1] Simon Watney spoke eloquently on behalf of the community of people who have or believe themselves to have HIV. He spoke of the need for trials established in collaboration with the communities affected by AIDS and HIV infection. He also spoke against the use of placebos (see pp. 173 ff. for glossary), and for the compelling need to remove the artificial (and at times brutal) distinction between research and treatment, and emphasized that the very reality of HIV disease impels us to offer treatment to people at many stages of HIV disease in a controlled research context. The other speaker was Dr Karen Gelmon, who is coordinating the trial in the United Kingdom. She spoke of the need for this trial, to see whether the development of AIDS can be prevented in people with HIV infection but without symptoms of severe disease. She spoke of the need for a placebo which, she insisted, is to ensure that we "don't come up with the wrong answer".

I attended the seminar as a double agent so to speak, because I am both a health educator with experience of statutory and non-statutory AIDS work, and a person living with HIV. Double agents are difficult for others to deal with because they go against the expectation that one's alter ego is kept out of sight. This can be particularly disconcerting for medical professionals who are socialized to expect medical encounters to reflect the role performance of doctor-professional or doctor-patient.[2] Like many people with HIV I am well informed about the subject. Of course we have a vested interest in keeping abreast of the issues, as the endlessly shifting terrain of social, cultural, scientific and political discourse frequently promises new disruptions to our civil liberties, our livelihoods, our mental and physical well-being and how we are perceived by others (and therefore in turn how we perceive ourselves). Like most other people, I wish to stay alive and well. I intend to die only when I have to, or when the pain of living is so great and the quality of my life is so impoverished that I take my life as a conscious act of choice. If it is at all possible, and reason as well as a growing body of knowledge suggests that it is, I would wish to prevent the development of more serious disease or that particular manifestation, which can result from infection with HIV, called AIDS.

I have had HIV for quite some time, probably since 1982, which is when I first developed Persistent Generalized Lymphadenopathy (PGL). I felt very ill that autumn with aches and chills, fevers and night sweats and a terrible sense of fatigue (which has never really gone away). This condition is now well documented and is considered to be an HIV sero-conversion illness, though at the time it did not exist as a disease entity at all. Therefore I could not really be ill; at least that is what my GP decided after first assuming (quite sensibly) that I probably had the "flu". He finally concluded, in response to my return visits complaining of continually aching glands, that it "was all in my mind". Later that year I visited St Mary's hospital "special clinic" in Praed Street because I was still concerned about my swollen glands: concerned because as a young gay man in the difficult process of coming out, and as a student of science, I had begun to read about AIDS. I was told by the physician that I couldn't possible have AIDS because he hadn't seen AIDS yet and was waiting for his first case. I didn't think I had AIDS but I knew I had something (glands, or lymph nodes, are not supposed to remain swollen) that might be related. The symptoms I had resembled the list of symptoms then typically described for AIDS, though they were all rather non-specific.

I mention this not to chart a tale of HIV and its lack of recognition by an uninformed medical profession, but to show that the "facts" about this medical entity have always been available as a mediator of experience only *retrospectively*. I have lived with a condition that at first did not exist. Then I was, along with countless others, "HIV antibody positive", which meant at first that only a minority of those infected would develop AIDS. Over the last few years we have lived with increasingly gloomy forecasts of progression rates. Germ theory has extended its ideological hold over AIDS knowledge, increasing causal determinacy to the point where we are increasingly told that most if not all of those infected with HIV will develop AIDS.

Clearly anyone with HIV would consider a treatment that offered the possibility of preventing the development of AIDS, particularly when told that without intervention they would die. Hence my personal interest in the proposed AZT (azdothymidine — brand name Zidovudine) trial. I had a further compelling reason. For much of the time with HIV I have been well, sometimes I have been ill, recently I have been quite ill. In fact I have been exhibiting observable symptoms, which is not only unpleasant (though there is a perverse pleasure in finally having something that a doctor can see) but has some unfortunate consequences. People can start behaving oddly if they know someone is HIV antibody positive. This oddness has got worse as people increasingly believe that HIV equals AIDS. One enters a vampiric state of the undead. It is a unique experience to know, whilst feeling very much alive, that one has entered the realm of the socially dead: the kingdom of the damned where one's destiny is a Hades-like world of silence, from which one is only able to pester the fully living with ghostly apparitions. This "social death" is a well observed phenomenon in all conditions perceived to be fatal. It does play on your mind and can lead to a sense of despair. So I went along to the seminar because I wanted to be seen to be living, and to voice my need to continue living to the doctors present (one wants to convince them first) as much as to learn about the trial and its restrictions.

The "Concorde 1" AZT trial is an Anglo-French initiative which aims to discover if the drug, which has been shown both to prolong life and to improve the condition of some people with AIDS,[3] will be successful in preventing the development of the syndrome in people with HIV. It is hoped that it will at least significantly delay the progression to more severe disease states.

The proposed method of research is as follows: one thousand people in the UK and a further thousand in France, all of whom have expressed a desire to take the drug will randomly be given either the drug or a placebo in the two "arms" of the trial. The trial will be "blinded" — which is to say that neither doctor nor patient knows if the patient is receiving the drug or the inert placebo. We were told by Dr Gelmon that the trial is needed to learn whether AZT is effective in preventing progressive HIV disease. In response to the question of whether the use of a placebo is ethical, we were told that it would be unethical to give everyone with HIV AZT because of the drug's toxicity.[4] In response to Simon Watney's point that a cohort of people (who strongly felt that they didn't want to take AZT) could be recruited from the gay community to act as a control, it was argued that there may be possible differences, either in the natural history of HIV or in drug action, between a group of people who would volunteer for a drug and a group who would not — thus producing an enhanced or diminished "placebo effect".

What became clear as the seminar progressed was the very real difference in priorities between the doctors present and the prospective participants. While both parties welcomed the dialogue, it was with quite different goals in mind. For the people with HIV and the AIDS workers present it was an opportunity to express unease about the trial, and to express needs for information, medical monitoring, and treatment options. For the medical profession, on the other hand, the seminar was seen as necessary to convince us of the need for this trial. Dr Ian Weller, the consultant who is chair of the MRC's working party for the trial said: "With AIDS, sharing information with patients has been absolutely critical to compliance ... it's inevitable in such a young population that they're going to be well informed."[5] It was instructive to see how the objections to the trial as proposed were refuted. The doctors rejected the use of laboratory markers which indicate the progress of HIV disease and the use of available preventive drug treatment for the most common infection in AIDS, Pneumocystis carinii Pneumonia (PCP). Indeed, all objections of a scientific nature were rejected on the grounds that there was no evidence to support them — along with the paternalistic reassurance that if any such convincing evidence for the effectiveness of new treatments were to emerge during the three year course of the trial, then, "of course," they would be used for the subjects' benefit.

That evening and in the days following I was not reassured. In fact, I was deeply distraught. How could such a calm assurance of the "self-evident" facts of the matter be maintained when things are clearly not so simple? A few days later, wandering down Oxford Street, I rather absent-mindedly took a magazine of the Hare Krishna order, *Back to Godhead*,[6] which contains a treatise called "Love and its Reflection" in which there is discussion of the character of absolute truth (Bhagavan) and how to realize it. There are many competing claims to absolute truth we are told, but only real absolute truth is replete with the six opulences: Beauty, Wealth, Strength, Fame, Knowledge, and Renunciation. These six opulences would be apparent in almost any representation of the modern doctor. The sexy, wealthy, medical detective renouncing all in the search for a cure, or the vigorous, handsome scientist-entrepreneur as hero are now common motifs. But what of knowledge? Surely scientific knowledge is made up of experimentally proven, objectively observable facts? Surely a fact just "is" and is not subject to ideological or cultural critique?

Scientific Models
Certainly scientific knowledge has been historically privileged. Until Kuhn,[7] most philosophies of science were defensive portraits of an idealized nineteenth-century positivist notion of science. Comparatively recently, however, developments in the history and philosophy of science, and the sociology of knowledge, have introduced a greater degree of relativism into the ways in which science is viewed, though this understanding has not yet entered the mainstream theory or practice of medicine.[8]

Science is not to be seen as basically positive or even as value neutral. Simple use/abuse, good science/bad science distinctions are similarly unhelpful. Accepting the ideological basis of science does not entail another dichotomy, ideology/truth, but means that science will necessarily reflect its historical precedents as well as the social values of its age.

In this context it is essential to see disease as a social construct. This is not to say that the biological "nature" of "AIDS" is determined by social concepts but that there are no straightforward facts of the matter. AIDS the concrete entity (whatever it may be) cannot be separated from "AIDS" the concept. The concept of a disease is socially and historically formed and psychologically and culturally embedded within a particular "thought style". Ludwik Fleck describes a thought style as:

The readiness for directed perception, with corresponding mental and objective assimilation of what has been so perceived. It is characterized by common features in the problems of interest to a thought collective, by the judgement which the thought collective considers evident, and by the methods which it applies as a means of cognition. The thought style may also be accompanied by a technical and literary style characteristic of the given system of knowledge. Because it belongs to a community, the thought style of the collective undergoes social reinforcement.[9]

A fact does not have self-evident being, it has a genesis and development. It emerges and is consolidated within a thought collective or stratified grouping of scientific practice. A fact becomes located within a thought style that is an interlocking frame of facts and knowledge which sociologically conditions that which is thought, as well as that which may not be debated.[10] As Barnes and Edge have stated of science in general:

> No body of knowledge, nor any part of one, can capture, or at least can be known to capture, *the* basic pattern or structure inherent in some aspect of the natural world. Nature can be patterned in different ways: it will tolerate many different orderings without protest, as is shown by the great variety of orderings which have been applied to it by experts, ancestors, aliens and deviants . . . Specific orderings are constructed not revealed, invented rather than discovered, in sequences of activity which however attentive to experience and to formal consistency could nonetheless have been otherwise and could have had different results. Hence in cleaving to its own specific body of knowledge a community commits itself to what is in an entirely non-pejorative sense, a system of conventions. Even the lowest-level formulations of the verbal culture of natural science, its statements of matters of fact and its recorded findings, have a conventional character.[11]

This mode of analysis is not just an abstract formulation that has little bearing on how things are really done in practice. It is crucial to an understanding of the principles on which the "Concorde 1" placebo controlled trial of AZT (Zidovudine) is based. It must be remembered that until recently the "cause" of AIDS was not understood. There were two main competing theories: immune-overload, and single agent theories.[12] It is not necessary to discuss these here, other than to point out that single-agent theory has won out. A consensus of medical and scientific opinion considers the Human Immunodeficiency Virus to be the "cause" of AIDS; its very name reveals its accepted aetiological role.

A reading of the popular "medical detective" stories of the discovery of the cause of AIDS will reveal the embellishments of the opulences of truth as a necessary part of "making a convincing case" for HIV as the cause of AIDS. Indeed Duesberg, a prominent virologist, has argued against HIV as the cause of AIDS. His arguments have at least shown that the pathogenesis (disease causing role) of HIV is not clearly understood.[13] Yet the point here is not to question that HIV is the "cause" of AIDS but to understand what the recognition of HIV as "cause" means and the significance of the location of "AIDS" within "germ-theory", which is so central to the thought-style of medical culture. This has certain inevitable consequences for medical practice around HIV and AIDS, in terms of the structure and function of research and treatment.

It is not an overstatement to say that modern medical science is built on germ-theory and its doctrine of specific aetiology. Indeed its most demonstrable therapeutic successes, "magic bullets" such as the invention of antibiotics, are the practical result of this theory. Classical germ-theory pictures a single agent as the cause of disease. There are also a number of principles known as Koch's postulates which have to be fulfilled to demonstrate the pathogenicity of a microbe. HIV has consistently failed to fulfil Koch's postulates.[14] This may be used to argue that HIV is not the cause of AIDS, but more importantly here, allowing that a theory is a model and not a "reflection" of truth, this failure demonstrates that the nineteenth-century germ-theory paradigm is inadequate to the task of explaining the complex aetiology of many diseases.

Yet clearly, germ-theory is the underlying principle of AIDS drug trials. HIV is seen as the specific agent; AIDS is the disease, manifested in the body; a potentially effective drug is seen as a would-be magic bullet, that is, a specific substance that can kill or incapacitate the single agent. The effectiveness of the trial (i.e. the success of the drug) is evaluated on the ability of the drug to stop, or prevent the emergence of, the disease in the treated subjects. However, this is an inadequate as well as a profoundly ideological logic. Just as germ-theory was seen by nineteenth-century science (and by and large still is) as ideologically neutral, so the body is seen as independent of ideology. As the bearer of organic disease, the object of study made manifest, the body is denied its social and cultural embodiment and comes to stand for the disease itself. Hence research on the body becomes legitimated; the body becomes the object of research (a kind of walk-in, skin-encapsulated test tube) and people become the legitimate subjects of research.

It is easy to see how the logic of drug trials demands the necessary use of human subjects as placebo arms, in whom the development of disease is allowed to develop unchecked; whilst in the drug treatment arm (one hopes), the disease will not develop or at least will be ameliorated. Here one can see why the end point for the non-treatment arm of the AZT trial must be severe (AIDS related) disease, the development of AIDS, or (AIDS related) death. According to the model, nothing else would convincingly demonstrate the effectiveness of the drug, or so we are told. Yet . . .

AIDS is Not a Disease

This must continually be asserted. The ideological consequence of the slippage between a syndrome and a disease has been stressed elsewhere in this volume; here it has crucial ideological and *aetiological* significance. In the history of disease, the process of recognition of new conditions usually starts with the epidemiological recognition of a syndrome. A syndrome is a set of signs and symptoms or a clustering that is useful for surveillance purposes. A syndrome is usually a set of distinct disease entities, each one of which may have distinct causes. The conventions of germ-theory attempt to resolve a syndrome in a linear manner, first into a single disease entity, and then into a single agent. Sometimes, as in the case of infectious disease, this can be done, although even here the causal determinacy of a single agent is not clear cut. *Mycobacterium tuberculis*, for instance, is a necessary but not sufficient cause of tuberculosis — since, if nutritional status is controlled, tuberculosis does not emerge. *Mycobacterium tuberculis* is in another sense not the cause of tuberculosis; it is the body's own immune response to the organism that causes tissue damage (i.e. the disease) rather than the direct action of the microbe. In many other conditions, causal determinacy is multifactorial (epidemiologists talk of a "web of causation"), and can involve many organismic and environmental contributions.[15]

AIDS is a syndrome. AIDS consists of many distinct diseases, infections and malignancies. Many are treatable and many preventable. The most common is Pneumocystis carinii Pneumonia (PCP) which accounts for over 60 per cent of AIDS diagnoses. It is highly preventable and yet the "Concorde 1" trial does not allow for prophylaxis (preventive treatment) for this condition (or for any other opportunistic infection).

The trial measures the effectiveness of the drug AZT by the appearance or non-appearance of AIDS in the non-treatment group compared to the treatment group. The naïvety of this approach (not to say its questionable ethical position) can be demonstrated if what we know of the causal picture of AIDS and its relationship to HIV is expanded to reflect a wider discourse of biomedicine that includes immunology and epidemiology as well as contemporary virology.

AIDS is a syndrome, a particular cluster of signs and symptoms that appears when a profound impairment of cell-mediated immunity takes place. This impairment is the result of long-standing infection with the Human Immunodeficiency Virus. The exact mechanism by which HIV achieves this damage is not known. In part, HIV appears to kill T-lymphocytes directly. Infected cells also seem able to attack other immune cells in a process of clumping known as syncytia.[16] Equally subtle but systematic deregulation of parts of the immune system take place via mechanisms that are as yet unclearly understood. Therefore, as in many other infections, part of the observable damage is likely to be due to the body's own immune response. Strictly speaking then, HIV is not the cause of AIDS. What it causes is the underlying immuno-suppression. Or, in other words, AIDS is not the disease but HIV associated immuno-suppression is.

An end-point for any therapeutic trial in HIV disease that consists of the emergence of opportunistic manifestations is thus not only unethical but also not scientifically logical. For if HIV associated immuno-suppression is the disease being treated, then therapeutic efficacy should be provable according to objective improvements in immune competence. Various measures exist in the form of laboratory blood-tests and clinical findings, that may provide direct evidence of immune function. In other cases, such indices also function as an evaluation of a person's current disease profile regarding HIV associated immuno-suppression, as well as representing prognostic indicators, or markers of disease progress and the likely onset of AIDS. It is perfectly possible, therefore, to construct well designed, controlled trials that are empirically sound, scientifically rational, and ethically acceptable. Yet there is an extraordinary inertia against doing so.

It may be argued that the resistance to redesigning therapeutic trials of interventions in HIV associated immuno-suppression is due to the machinations of drug companies who have a financial stake in the current structure and funding of trials. The market system puts a real premium on researching a novel (and therefore more easily patentable) substance, in preference to an existing substance that is cheap and harmless but unpatentable.[17] The penetration and control of drug companies into all aspects of modern biomedical research, from academic university departments to clinical research in hospitals and general practitioners' surgeries, is not to be underestimated.[18] However, what is being argued here is not a general conspiracy theory of research, or even, in an individualist sense, of particular researchers.

In a very real sense AIDS and HIV are social and technological constructs. Yet they are also constructs of late twentieth-century techniques of virology and immunology, and have emerged in an epistemological hiatus where the theoretical formulations of the germ-theory paradigm are inadequate to the task of explaining the existence let alone the pathogenicity of HIV. A paradigmatic bulge has occurred that could generate new ways of thinking and practice in relationship to viruses in particular and disease mechanisms in general. A theory of thought-styles and thought-collectives would however lead us to be more cautious before announcing the emergence of a new paradigm (that is a better model of truth than its predecessors). Thought-styles are cognitive halters that are produced socially and culturally within a collective of self-referring experts. The conditions of credibility of knowledge are therefore quite literally formed in social spaces (hospitals, laboratories, commonrooms, conferences and dinner parties) where the mode of practice of experts is constituted.[19] The model of the effective drug trial is caught firmly within a nineteenth-century paradigm. A theory of thought-styles allows us to see that the Kuhnian notion of a paradigm as an intellectual pattern or exemplar, does not fully explain the manner in which knowledge is tenaciously reproduced.

Persuasive, believable, credible knowledge is directed psychologically, culturally, and historically, within thought-collectives, in this instance from within the actual institutions and social worlds of AIDS doctors and researchers.[20]

All well and good you might say, but how on earth does anyone set about changing this state of affairs? From the above critique two possibilities present themselves. The first is to engage in an educational programme for physicians and researchers to convince them of the existence of a paradigm shift and the need for theoretical reformulations of existing knowledge based on an intense reading in the history and philosophy of science, the sociology of knowledge, cultural studies and ideology critique. Not a particularly likely prospect. The other option is to find or construct a social and theoretical space where the possibilities of research and treatment can be thought differently. Such a "window of opportunity" does in fact currently present itself: the Community Research Initiative (CRI).

Community Research Initiatives

In the United States in late 1986, the New York Community Research Initiative came into being as a grassroots initiative by the People With AIDS Coalition, conceived of and first set up by Dr Joseph Sonnabend and Michael Callen among others.[21] In its original form it represented little more than a new recruitment strategy, utilizing the private physicians of people with HIV associated immuno-suppression in the New York area, though community workers with ideals of community empowerment and participation soon became involved. It also differed from conventional drug research in proposing interventions of promising therapies prior to the emergence of AIDS in the hope of halting disease progression.

Since then, community research initiatives or community research alliances (a Californian term) have sprung up in many urban areas in the United States and are now being developed in Britain. A CRI certainly sounds good but does it actually offer the promise of better research and treatment? Again that depends very much on what one's model of a community and of research is. Several very clear tensions seem to be apparent in the movement, or rather two issues around which opinion tends to polarize.

The first issue is that of deregulation, which in effect is what a CRI (in attempting to expedite research by circumventing the large bureaucratic multi-centre trials) represents. At one end of the spectrum of opinion are the radical deregulators, who represent the interests of the drug companies and the therapeutics market (both orthodox and alternative). Certainly CRI's have often found it difficult to raise funds for research into cheap substances that have little current scientific credibility; they increasingly find themselves approached by drug companies (who also have an interest in less regulated research), often with offers that are difficult to refuse.[22] Clearly CRI's are not perceived as an inherent threat to the existing structure of medical research. For example, Dr Frank Young of the US Food and Drug Administration (FDA) was able in July 1988 to announce the incorporation of CRI's into the system of licensing and approval of drugs.[23] At the other end of the deregulation spectrum lies a series of concerns for community empowerment and participation that come out of the tradition of the cultural critique of statist medicine as exemplified by black community groups, feminists, radical psychotherapists, and health policy analysts.[24]

The second issue is that of care and treatment versus research. The ethical and practical difficulties of this conflict are intrinsic to much of this article, and the issues they raise are further discussed in the glossary. However this will become a particularly fraught issue for CRI's, as they could just become community recruitment initiatives for the kind of research that necessitated their coming into being in the first place. Put simply, the drug researcher is not primarily concerned with providing optimal care for individual subjects, and research (as presently conducted) is not likely to produce the best patient management strategies. It is critical to recognize that good management strategies are life prolonging. As Dr Joseph Sonnabend writes:

> People with AIDS die from well recognized opportunistic manifestations. Opportunistic infections can sometimes be prevented, are frequently treatable and can sometimes be detected by tests before clinical disease develops.[25]

As stated elsewhere it cannot therefore be ethical to withhold life prolonging therapies in the interest of research.

GLOSSARY

Accrual

The procedure of recruiting people to be the subjects of therapeutic trials. Large-scale randomized controlled trials typically have very low accrual rates. This is not surprising given the ambiguous motives of such trials. If a doctor cannot know whether the intervention will prove effective, or even whether the subject will receive it or a placebo, reticence on the part of the subject is an understandable response. Researchers often seek ways to get round their ethical duty to provide treatment. They therefore tend to use "pre-selection" or "pre-randomization" before entering subjects into trials. This means that trials can never be truly random as some selection bias is inevitable, not least because by the very act of volunteering a subject group ceases to be a random sample.[26]

Community

Throughout the literature of AIDS we encounter groups of people who are routinely described as communities. These include "the haemophiliac community", "the gay community" and, increasingly, "the heterosexual community". It is however far from clear what such groups have in common. In this context the notion of community serves the ideological purpose of erasing structural inequalities, and implies that any group of people categorized as a community is inherently autonomous and politically equal. Use of the term "community" should be retained to designate a site of collectivity distinct from the larger society in which it resides. The description of dominant society, white, heterosexual, ruling-class, as a series of "communities" only serves to reinforce the hegemony of these groups. From a liberation perspective, community research or community education would involve participation in and empowerment of the community, rather than one section of society being a subject of research or education. Such an approach recognizes that communities are not necessarily pre-given but are often forged through the collective experience of oppression to which they respond.[27]

Compliance

The degree of (patient) conformity to the conditions of treatment or a therapeutic trial. Prior to the emergence of modern, demonstrably effective therapeutics, there was little sustained concern over whether patients took their drugs or not. This changed with the age of antibiotics when an individualistic approach in the new field of medical sociology became concerned with "uncooperative patients". It was believed that certain personality characteristics were responsible for poor compliance. It was also believed that research would lead to the identification of "unreliable patients" so that appropriate remedial measures could be taken. Since the sixties however, interactive analyses have developed that look at communication between doctor, patient and significant others in the health system. Blackwell found that in a review of over fifty studies, between 25 and 50 per cent of outpatients completely failed to take their medication. As he stated: "The most important contribution to compliance is the understanding a patient has of the illness, the need for treatment, and the likely consequences of both. Time spent in explaining these issues pays multiple dividends, not least in the sense of alliance that emerges when patient and physician believe they are collaborating."[28] It is worth asking to what extent participants may believe they are collaborating if they know they are being denied potentially life-prolonging treatments. One alternative to randomly assigned placebo groups that has been suggested is that a group of people who do not wish to take the drug be recruited through the community to serve as a control. The argument against this is always that there may be significant differences in the two groups that may have a bearing on their health. Such differences, however, would have to be ones that stand a reasonable chance of having some effect, diet or stress reduction for instance. Presumably one cannot prevent trial participants from also taking dietary therapies or medication. Yet as a serious cost benefit calculation, it is reasonable to assume that one would get better results from recruiting those people who genuinely want the drug (who else would volunteer?) and actually giving it to them, thereby ensuring higher "compliance" rates.

Consent (Informed)

Principle 9 of the Declaration of Helsinki (revised 1975 and 1983) states: "In any research on human beings, each potential subject must be adequately informed of the aims, methods, anticipated benefits and potential hazards of the study and the discomfort it may entail. He or she should be informed that he or she is at liberty to abstain from participation in the study and that he or she is free to withdraw his or her consent to participation at any time. The doctor should then obtain the subject's freely given informed consent, preferably." Article 10 states that: "When obtaining informed consent for the research project the doctor should be particularly cautious if the subject is in a dependent relationship to him or her or may consent under duress. In that case the informed consent should be obtained by a doctor who is not engaged in the investigation and who is completely independent of this official relationship."[29]

Unfortunately informed consent is not a concept endorsed by British law or by the culture of medical practice, although the British Medical Association endorses the principle. The status of informed consent for people with HIV, especially those newly diagnosed, is highly problematic since informed consent should involve access to information regarding one's current health status. This should include laboratory findings that are well known prognostic indicators, together with frank discussion of their significance in terms of their ability to predict the probability of severe disease.

Controlled Trials
The model of a controlled trial is very simple. In order to find out whether a new treatment is better than an existing one, or no treatment at all, the new intervention is given to a group of patients, or healthy volunteers, and denied to another group chosen to be as similar as possible. However it is the intricacy of trial design that is critical for its success. The essential problem is that a treatment of relatively unknown safety and efficacy is given to one group; or putting this another way, a potentially promising treatment is given to one group. This means that the non-treatment group may have had improved health had they not been restricted by the conditions of the trial. A trial must provide an answer as quickly as possible, and must be stopped as soon as demonstrably harmful effects occur. Controlled trials are further controlled by the techniques of double-blinding and randomization. Double-blind trials are set up to eliminate the subjective tendency for doctors to have a preference in treatment. The technique keeps the choice of treatment, or no treatment at all, secret from both the doctor and the patient. This means that the patient's doctor cannot be a researcher on the trial.[30] It also means that the patient's doctor must agree to the ethics of the trials protocol. In the case of AZT (Zidovudine) trials, double-

blinding is almost impossible. Due to the drug's characteristic effects on laboratory indices such as the "mean corpuscular volume", any physician would be rapidly able to tell if a subject were on the drug. The attempt to get round this is to blind or "hide" these results from the subject's doctors and the subjects themselves. Not only is this profoundly unethical, it is potentially harmful, as the drug AZT has well known toxicities, information about which would have to be hidden in order to keep the trial blinded. The participating centres of the Concorde 1 trial by definition have the greatest clinical knowledge of dealing with HIV. People entering the trial in such centres will expect the same standard of care, information, and honesty as non-trial people in the same centre. The very nature of the trial conditions however, cuts across the ethically proper patient/doctor relationship. The protocols of this trial, by making AZT the only drug permissible, deny the use of prophylaxis for various opportunistic infections. Yet prophylaxis is de facto a fundamental aspect of correct and ethical patient management.

Disease, Illness and Sickness

A consensus in medical sociology distinguishes between disease, illness and sickness. Disease is the organic biomedically defined disorder. Illness is the subjective experience of ill-health. Sickness becomes the social projection of ill-health or the social "sick-role". The trouble with this convenient distinction is that it lets the category of disease off the hook, by privileging it as a value neutral series of facts that exist in nature. As Turner points out,[31] this implies a division between mind and body, as well as reflecting the professional disciplines of medicine (disease), psychology (illness) and medical sociology (sickness). However, in the context of the placebo trial this tripartite distinction serves the useful function of pointing out that taking a placebo four times a day for up to three years can make a person ill, and socially sick (irrespective of any underlying disease) when they may not have been at the outset.

Ethics of Human Research

The widespread sense of horror that followed the revelation of mass medical experimentation conducted by doctors in the concentration camps in Nazi occupied Europe led to the first internationally agreed statement governing human biomedical research — the Nuremberg Code. The medical profession however did not publicly endorse its principles until the Declaration of Helsinki was drawn up by the World Medical Association in 1964 (subsequently revised in 1975 and 1983). In Britain the Medical Research Council (MRC) produces an advisory document on research entitled, "Responsibility in Investigation on Human Subjects 1962". There is in fact an inherent conflict expressed throughout international codes governing research on human subjects between the ethical duties of the primary care physician and the medical researcher. We can nonetheless distinguish two types of research on humans.

Medical research combined with professional care (clinical research); and non-therapeutic biomedical research involving human subjects (non-clinical biomedical research). The MRC AIDS directed programme consists entirely of a portfolio of non-clinical research. There were no concrete plans for a directed clinical research trial. The money for the Concorde 1 trial has come from existing financial arrangements.

Whilst it is unethical to conduct research that is badly designed or inadequately executed, it does not follow that well planned and conducted research is necessarily ethical. The ethics of human experimentation should always be governed by principles other than scientific merit alone. Controlled clinical trials should always be approved by a properly constituted external ethical committee. Unfortunately such committees have a low profile in British medical culture. They publish neither proceedings nor reports, and in many instances do not even meet. Yet in the United States they wield a great deal of power and are required by federal law to have lay representatives, whilst their power extends to cover therapeutic and prognostic matters. In Britain, there seems to be a clear case for governmental guidance, or even direction.[32]

Placebo

A chemically inert substance, forming the intervention for the non-treatment arm of a placebo controlled trial. A placebo is usually designed to look like the drug for which it is substituted. It therefore involves deceiving the subject. This involves complex moral issues. On the one hand the trial drug may be very harmful and/or inefficacious, in which case only half of the trial group is being harmed. On the other hand the placebo group may be denied access to a beneficial treatment. Both groups may be denied other contingent forms of treatment. The use of placebos is difficult to justify ethically, though they have scientific merit in some circumstances. Their use should always be carefully controlled. It is the ethical responsibility of research to state precisely why a trial cannot be conducted in any other way. Placebos can only be justified when there is no alternative, for example when there is no genuine alternative to the experimental drug.[33] AZT is the only drug approved for usage in AIDS. However there are scores of existing substances under investigation in other countries which show promise and yet are not being researched in this country. Thus claims that placebos are justified because there is no known alternative treatment can only be sustained by the failure to conduct trials of other drugs. It is also difficult to sustain the argument that a placebo is necessary because there is no "cure" for AIDS, when it is known that proper patient management is critical to patient survival time. A placebo trial can not avoid interfering with the prompt diagnosis, and early and aggressive intervention required to keep people alive. Strictly speaking, people do not die of AIDS, but of opportunistic conditions, many of which are treatable or preventable. In the United States 15 per cent of people with AIDS live for up to five years;[34] they clearly wouldn't do so if placed on a placebo trial and hence denied the full benefits of treatment.

Laboratory Markers

There are many laboratory markers that are meaningful in HIV associated immuno-suppression and four are gaining credibility as predictive of progression to AIDS:

CD4 (or T4) Lymphocyte count. Normal ranges are absolute counts of 800–900. Most people with HIV remain without symptoms for several years after infection, with counts greater than 400. Over three years approximately 14 per cent progress to AIDS. About 50 per cent of people without symptoms but counts lower than 400 develop AIDS in three years. About 90 per cent of people with symptoms and fewer than 400 CD4 lymphocytes progress to AIDS in the same time. A single T cell count is difficult to interpret but a very low count or a consistently downward trend is significant.

Antigen test. A test for HIV p24 core antigen (a virus particle in the centre of HIV). This antigen is usually present just after someone has been infected with HIV. Then it disappears but may appear again later. In some people it remains present and they are likely to develop AIDS quite rapidly. This test can be combined with the T cell count for greater predictive value. Approximately 45 per cent of people with a CD4 count of more than 400 and a positive antigen test will progress to AIDS in three years. Below 400 and a positive antigen test gives an 80 per cent probability of developing AIDS.

B-2 Microglobulin is a protein that seems to be released from the surface of some cells of the immune system. The normal value of B-2 microglobulin is 1.7. About 25 per cent of people with CD4 counts higher than 400 and B-2 count of greater than three will develop AIDS in three years. People with similar B-2 counts and lower than 400 CD4 lymphocytes have up to a 75 per cent probability chance of developing AIDS over three years.

Neopterin is a protein produced from macrophages (an immune cell that plays an important role in HIV). Neopterin counts seem to correlate well with B–2 microglobulin counts and seem to have similar predictive properties.

All of this information comes from an article by Andrew Moss, a British epidemiologist based at San Francisco General Hospital[35] who concludes that these tests should be "explored for their usefulness in stratifying subjects for trials for treatment and as measures of outcome". Sadly none of these tests are routine for the vast majority of people who know they are infected with HIV, but for the most part lack any regular monitoring. How can people be expected to give informed consent to a placebo trial that is intended to run for three years when information that is predictive over three years is denied?

Postscript
Within a week of attending the Concorde-1 Seminar in Earls Court, I left one hospital that denied me the information from laboratory markers yet offered me the placebo trial and went to another hospital where, on the basis of laboratory indicators and clinical findings, I was offered AZT directly.

Notes

1. D. Campbell, "AIDS patient puts research on trial", *New Scientist*, 12 November 1988.

2. see, for example, T. Parsons, *The Social System*, New York 1951 and Erving Goffman, *Asylums*, New York 1961.

3. M. Fischl et. al., "The efficacy of Azdothymidine (AZT) in the treatment of patients with AIDS and AIDS related complex", *New England Journal of Medicine*, no. 317, pp. 185–91.

4. D.D. Richman, "The toxicity of Azdothymidine (AZT) in the treatment of patients with AIDS and AIDS related complex", *New England Journal of Medicine*, no. 317, pp. 192–7.

5. Campbell, op.cit., p. 26.

6. A.C. Bhaktivedenta, "Love and Its Reflection", in *Back to Godhead*, London 1988.

7. T. Kuhn, *The Structure of Scientific Revolutions*, Chicago 1970.

8. For an introduction to the philosophy of science, see A.F. Chalmers, *What is This Thing Called Science*, Milton Keynes 1982; Paul Feyerabend, *Against Method*, London 1978. For a sociology of knowledge perspective, see P. Berger and T. Luckman, *The Social Construction of Reality*, Harmondsworth 1971

9. L. Fleck, *Genesis and Development of a Scientific Fact*, Chicago 1979, p. 99.

10. M. Horton and P. Aggleton, "Perverts, Inverts and Experts: The cultural production of an AIDS research paradigm" in Aggleton, Hart and Davies (eds.) *AIDS Social Representations*, London 1989.

11. B. Barnes and D. Edge, *Science in Context*, Oxford 1982.

12. E. Johnson and P. Ho, "The Elusive Etiology of AIDS", in V. G Gong, *Understanding AIDS*, New Brunswick 1985.

13. Moss et al, *Science*, November 1988. See also J. Lauritsen, "Saying no to HIV", *New York Native*, 6 July 1987. An interview with Professor Peter Duesberg (the man who discovered the genetic sequencing of HIV and a prominent virologist who claims that HIV is not the cause of AIDS).

14. J. Lauritsen, *New York Native*, 27 October 1986.

15. B. McMahon and T.F. Pugh, *Epidemiology Principles and Methods*, Boston, MA 1970. For a marxist analysis of the causes of ill health, see L. Doyal, *The Political Economy of Health*, London 1979.

16. see *Scientific American*, October 1988 for current thinking on the pathogenicity of HIV infection.

17. D. Campbell, "The AIDS Scam", *New Statesmen & Society*, 24 June 1988.

18. See the "MRC AIDS directed" programme document for an idea of the level of collaboration between commercial companies and even basic AIDS research.

19. M. Horton and P. Aggleton, op. cit., L. Fleck, op. cit.

20. M. Horton and P. Aggelton, op. cit., for an idea of how these thought-structures might operate in AIDS knowledge formation.

21. Joseph Sonnabend, Michael Callen et al, "Community Research Initiatives; A proposal for the prevention of AIDS", PWA coalition New York, 12 November 1986; see also, Simon Watney, "Catastrophic Rights", *Gay Times*, no. 115, February 1989, and Simon Watney, "Early intervention research gets started", *Capital Gay*, no. 378, 3 February 1989.

22. Joseph Sonnabend, personal communication.

23. Dr Frank Young of the US Food and Drug Agency, Address to the International Lesbian and Gay Health Conference, Boston July 1988.

24. J. Ehrenreich, *The Cultural Crisis of Modern Medicine*, New York 1977, for a review of this.

25. J. Sonnabend in Michael Callen (ed.), *AIDS Forum*, no. 1, New York 1989.

26. J. K. Mason and R.A. Smith McCall, *Law and Medical Ethics*, London 1987.

27. P. Freire, *Pedagogy of the Oppressed*, Harmondsworth 1978.

28. B. Blackwell, cited in B. Barber, *Informed Consent in Medical Therapy and Research*, New Brunswick 1980, p. 90.

29. Mason and McCall in Smith, op. cit.

30. Ibid.

31. B. S. Turner, *Medical Power and Social Knowledge*, London 1987.

32. Mason and McCall, in Smith, op. cit., p. 257.

33. Ibid.

34. R. Rothenberg et al, *New England Journal of Medicine*, no. 297.

35. A. Moss, "Predicting Who Will Progress to AIDS", *British Medical Journal*, no. 297, pp. 1067-8.

SIMON WATNEY

AIDS, LANGUAGE AND THE THIRD WORLD

Introduction
Language plays a central role in determining public perceptions of
all aspects of AIDS, and its many consequences around the world.
Language shapes attitudes and beliefs, which in turn inform
behaviour. Sadly, a number of fundamental misconceptions about
AIDS are still widespread in the United Kingdom. These include
notions concerning the syndrome itself, who is at risk, and what can
be done to protect people. The Declaration which concluded the
London World AIDS Summit in January 1988 emphasized, "the need
in AIDS prevention programmes to protect human rights and human
dignity". Unfortunately this has not always been achieved. This is
especially evident in the reporting of AIDS in the Third World, which
is frequently regarded as if it were somehow to blame for the entire
global epidemic. We therefore need to be specially careful whenever
we write about any aspect of HIV or AIDS. This is in all our interests,
since ignorance and prejudice have long proved to be the
staunchest friends of infectious diseases. All too often AIDS is
presented as if it were someone else's problem. It is however vitally
important that everyone should recognize that AIDS is a global
disaster, and that we are all involved in it together. It is also
important to emphasize that we are not powerless in relation to AIDS.
We can help one another as individuals, as communities, and as
nations.

Since much misunderstanding derives from the reporting of
medical information, it is first necessary to define and distinguish
HIV and AIDS.

HIV and AIDS

AIDS stands for the Acquired Immune Deficiency Syndrome, a set of medically defined conditions first identified in the United States in the early 1980s. AIDS is not a disease as such, but a collection of many different medical conditions including infections, cancers and tumours, which may emerge as the result of damage to the body's immunological defences caused by the Human Immunodeficiency Virus (HIV). Much has been learned about the natural history of HIV since its isolation in 1983, and its modes of transmission are well established. Yet the confidence which should derive from this knowledge is often undermined by careless, or ill-informed reporting. It is most important to avoid such inaccuracies since they may confuse readers, or reinforce unrealistic and unfounded fears, or encourage complacency. There are at least five major areas to consider:

1. Contagion Versus Infection. Whilst HIV is infectious in a limited number of circumstances, it is *not* a contagious condition. It cannot be "caught" like the common cold. All terms which imply contagion, such as "spreading" or "catching" should be rejected. AIDS of course is neither infectious nor contagious, since its various symptoms are direct results of previous HIV infection. The Centers for Disease Control (CDC) in Atlanta, Georgia, now calculate an average period of eight years between infection by HIV, and an AIDS diagnosis. It should therefore be apparent that nobody "catches" AIDS, since it is not a single condition. Furthermore, the various conditions which are collectively classified as AIDS may appear in a wide variety of sequences and combinations. These differ according to the many variations in individual health, the prevalence of different viruses and bacteria around the world to which people with HIV may become vulnerable, and other factors. In all of this it is important to understand that AIDS is experienced in a wide variety of ways by different people. In this context it should also be apparent that the notion of so-called "AIDS carriers" is particularly misleading, since it confuses HIV and AIDS, and manages to imply that *both* are contagious conditions.

2. Risk Factors. Epidemiologists, who study the distribution and changing patterns of disease, sometimes refer to "high-risk groups". This is intended to identify groups that have proved vulnerable to a given medical problem, in order to secure and direct appropriate resources, which may vary from drugs, to vaccines, or health education. Degrees of risk are very rarely innate, or fixed, and tend to vary over time. By describing the social groups who were first affected by HIV as "high-risk groups", the implication may be incorrectly established that other people are *not* at risk. With HIV it cannot be sufficiently emphasized that risk comes from what you do, not how you label yourself. There is no *intrinsic* relation between HIV and any individual or population group. It is therefore advisable to refrain from using the term "high-risk groups" unless one is writing for a specialist audience. What should be stressed are *risk factors*. These include the sharing of syringes, and unprotected sexual intercourse. Yet even risk factors may change. For example, the number of one's sexual partners was a risk factor before the existence of HIV was known or even suspected. Now that gay men practice Safer Sex, the number of their sexual partners is not a significant risk factor.

3. Victimization. One of the most important aspects of the experience of all diseases is the degree of control that affected individuals are able to exercise in their everyday lives. AIDS is no exception to this rule. On the contrary, since most people with HIV lead active and productive lives it is important that they should not be burdened with the deeply misleading label of "victims". People with AIDS may be victimized by prejudice or ignorance or direct discrimination from other people and institutions, but they themselves face the same choices concerning all aspects of their lives as everybody else. The majority of people with AIDS spend less than 20 per cent of their lives in hospital after diagnosis, and we should respect their refusal to see themselves as "victims", as if they were entirely passive and powerless.

4. Testing. Much misunderstanding about HIV and AIDS derives from continued reference to the so-called "AIDS virus". This term obscures the crucial distinction between HIV and AIDS, and confuses many people. We should always take the trouble to distinguish clearly between the two, not least in order to do justice to the lived experience of people with HIV and people with AIDS. The notion of the "AIDS virus" also lends credibility to the equally misleading notion of the so-called "AIDS test". It should be pointed out that the most widely used test for indicating HIV infection detects the presence or absence of antibodies in the blood produced in response to the virus. It should always be referred to accurately as the HIV antibody test. Besides, how could one test possibly be sensitive to all the conditions collectively known as AIDS, as well as antibodies to the virus? One cannot test for a syndrome, which is a medical category, not a single disease.

5. Life Expectancy. Many accounts of AIDS unfortunately imply that it is more or less instantly fatal. This entirely obscures the fact that there are many long-term survivors of the syndrome, who have lived with AIDS for more than five years. The imagery of 100 per cent fatality does nothing to help the thousands of people living with AIDS. It also overlooks the fact that although most people with AIDS have died within a few years of diagnosis, we do not know for sure that everyone with the syndrome will die as a result. Life expectancy has improved dramatically for many people with AIDS as a result of drug treatments and prophylactics against individual diseases characteristic of AIDS. Since these "opportunistic conditions" may arise in such a wide variety of sequences and combinations, there is no single or typical experience of the syndrome. The frequent emphasis on death in AIDS commentary is at best sentimental, and at worst simply morbid.

AIDS and the Third World

It is always important to recognize that every country affected by HIV has its own epidemic, shaped by the local circumstances of the population groups in which the virus first emerges. This is not to say that HIV is a different disease in different countries, but that the patterns of its transmission are profoundly influenced by social context. World Health Organization statistics demonstrate that HIV has had a disproportionate impact in the developing world, including Africa, the Caribbean, and South and Latin America. It has also had a disproportionate impact among people of colour in the United States, where 40 per cent of cases are found among blacks and Hispanics, who make up only 19 per cent of the overall population.

It is clear that countries as far apart as Brazil, Tanzania, Mexico, Bermuda and Haiti have epidemics as serious as those in Europe.

Comparisons between different epidemics should not be based on numbers of cases, but on the ratio of cases to the national population as a whole. Thus, whilst Haiti and Britain have approximately the same number of cases, the proportion of people with AIDS in Haiti is five times that in the UK. It is not surprising that the situation of most people with AIDS faithfully reflects their social and economic position *before* they contracted HIV. This is cruelly apparent from life expectancy statistics, which reveal that a white American man lives on average some three or four times longer with AIDS than a black American woman. Such figures indicate relative access to expensive drugs, health education, and general health care provision.

We should also recognize that whereas the average ratio of men to women with AIDS in Europe and the USA is 16:1, in some African countries it is 1:1. This alerts us to the fact that in many parts of the world, unprotected heterosexual intercourse is by far the most significant risk factor in the transmission of HIV. We are all familiar with the types of argument that present AIDS in Kenya or Uganda as "special cases", with attempts to "explain" their epidemics in a wide variety of exotic ways, ranging from ritual scarring to supposed bestiality, with frequent reference to the scientifically discredited Green Monkey hypothesis. Yet as long ago as 1985, researchers from the London Institute of Cancer Research investigated and ruled out all other significant factors in the transmission of HIV in Africa — except unprotected heterosexual intercourse.

As Cindy Patton has pointed out: "The unconscious belief that a strange new virus could not have arisen from the germ-free West led researchers on a fantastic voyage in search of the origins of HIV first in Haiti and then in Africa." In this context it is important to recognize that there is no conclusive evidence concerning the origins of HIV, and many epidemiologists reject the idea that it appeared first in Africa. It seems unlikely that we will ever know for sure where the virus originated, but even if we did, we should not make the foolish mistake of blaming the people of that unknown locality. We must constantly be on our guard against attempts to blame the different social and racial groups affected first by HIV as if they were somehow its *cause*. The unfortunate tendency to blame AIDS on the Third World only adds racial insult to the tragic injuries of disease and human suffering.

This is especially the case in relation to the reporting of HIV and

AIDS in Africa, which is all too often treated as if it were a single country, without the cultural, religious, ethnic and economic variations that are taken for granted in Europe or the USA. At the same time we frequently read of the "AIDS riddled" cities of Kinshasa or Nairobi, whereas Western cities such as London or Paris are merely "affected", or at worst "devastated", which at least suggests some implication of tragedy and human sympathies. In a similar manner, we read of "AIDS infested" prostitutes in Africa, with the strong implication that African women are unclean, and that AIDS may be transmitted via insects such as lice, for which the term "infestation" is generally reserved. On the one hand we are informed that any unmarried African woman having sex is a "prostitute", and supposedly a deadly threat, while on the other, black African women's lives would appear to be completely unvalued, and their vital role as potential Safer Sex educators is ignored. Such reporting tells us far more about the beliefs and attitudes of white journalists, than about the complex realities of AIDS. It seems likely that the relentless emphasis on supposed African "promiscuity" is one way of avoiding the diversity and complexity of human sexuality in all countries. It also conveniently obscures the widespread disruption of social life in many African nations as the result of economic exploitation by the West, and their long struggles for independence.

In a similar fashion, African countries are frequently blamed for under-reporting HIV and AIDS statistics, as if such figures were easily available in any society, as if under-reporting is not as frequent in the USA or Britain as it is in Uganda or Zaire. The major problem confronting those working in AIDS education throughout the developing world is that of resources, a problem which is only worsened by misreporting in the West, which represents AIDS in other parts of the world as if it were inevitable and unpreventable. In this context, a number of separate issues need to be raised:

1. **Immigration and HIV Antibody Testing.** The Report of the World Health Organization's Consultation on International Travel and HIV Infection (Geneva, March 1987), concluded that: "HIV screening programmes for international travellers would, at best and at *great* cost, retard *only briefly* the dissemination of HIV both globally and with respect to any particularly country." Sadly, the delusion that everyone with HIV can be identified, and the epidemic halted in its

tracks, is still not uncommon. It may result on the one hand in the unjustified HIV antibody testing of Third World citizens visiting First and Second World countries; and on the other it has led countries such as India to introduce similar measures directed for example at black African students, but not at American or British tourists. In the absence of either a cure for HIV infection, or a vaccine against it, the only effective measures to prevent the further transmission of the virus remain health education and Safer Sex. Monogamy may slow down the rate of transmission in some circumstances, but it is of course no guarantee that one or both partners is not already infected. In short, we cannot test or legislate HIV out of existence.

2. Discrimination and Human Rights. We have already encountered examples of reporting where racial prejudice skews judgement and leads to distorted attitudes and policies. HIV is not a property of persons, and although it is very prevalent in some parts of the Third World, it is dangerous simply to regard it as a disease of poverty. As Cindy Patton points out, such a description only reinforces the mistaken assumption that, "the lack of Western-style industrialization, rather than a virus, causes AIDS in Africa." In May 1988 the World Health Organization's World Health Assembly in Geneva adopted resolution WHA41.24 which urges Member States: "to foster a spirit of understanding and compassion for HIV infected people and people with AIDS through information and social support programmes" and to "avoid discriminatory measures against and stigmatization of them in the provision of services, employment and travel." The resolution also requests the Director General: "to stress to member states and to all others the dangers to the health of everyone of discriminatory action against and stigmatization of HIV infected people and people with AIDS.".

3. Risk Factors, Patient Care and Patients' Rights. The risk factors for HIV infection throughout the developing world are very clear: they are unprotected sexual intercourse, whether anal or vaginal, the sharing of needles and syringes by injecting drug users, and the possibility of infected blood entering blood banks. All three areas can be remedied — given adequate resources in the form of effective AIDS education; the provision of needle-exchange projects and education for injecting drug users on the possible risk to their sexual partners; and blood screening procedures for all blood banks. Such measures are being implemented throughout the Third World, with support from the World Health Organization and many other national and international institutions. In such circumstances we might contrast the regrettable spectacle of thousands of homeless people with AIDS living rough in shelters in the USA, to the example of care and love in the worst affected regions of Central and Eastern Africa. One factor which has given rise to concern and controversy is that of breast feeding. In June 1987 the Special Programme on AIDS of the World Health Organization concluded that: "Breast feeding should continue to be promoted in both developing and developed countries" since "the overall immuno-logical, nutritional, psychosocial and child-spacing benefits of breast feeding to infants and their mothers continue to be important factors in determining the overall health of mother and child." There is a substantially greater risk to health from artificial feeding than from the remote possibility of HIV transmission during breast feeding.

Conclusion

Sander Gilman has observed that: "It is the fear of collapse, the sense of dissolution, which contaminates the Western image of all diseases . . . But the fear we have of our own collapse does not remain internalized. Rather, we project this fear onto the world in order to localize it and, indeed, to domesticate it. For once we locate it, the fear of our own dissolution is removed. Then it is not we who totter on the brink of collapse, but rather the Other. And it is an-Other who has already shown his or her vulnerability by having collapsed."[2] Western commentary on AIDS in the Third World tells us much about the forms of contemporary racism. Thus, while AIDS in Africa is generally regarded as intrinsically different from AIDS in Europe, this does not prevent French virologists from conducting vaccine experiments on soldiers from the Zaire army.

From such contradictions we learn that disease continues to play a major role in constructing powerful symbolic boundaries, which define the identities of individuals, communities, and nations. For many centuries Western colonialism attempted to justify the exploitation of Third World peoples by a series of analogies which presented blacks and people of colour as "naturally" submissive, inferior, fit only to provide labour for their white masters. Yet it was always at the same time evident that "the natives" were physically stronger and more resilient in the face of disease than the white colonialists. Hence the shift to a racism rooted in late nineteenth century notions concerning the supposedly innate differences of intelligence between races. It seems that Western AIDS commentary will go to any lengths to obscure the fact that HIV is simply a virus, to which we are all potentially vulnerable. Hence the relentless demonizing of all the communities around the world that have been most devastated by AIDS.[3]

Yet the West can learn much from the experience of these communities, if it were only prepared to listen. As the head of Uganda's national AIDS prevention committee explains: "There is a snake in the house. Do you just sit and ask where the snake came from? Should we not be more concerned with what action needs to be taken now that the snake is in the house?"[4] Whilst Western governments launch punitive legislation and moral invectives against the very communities that are most in need of support in these times, and collude with ugly discrimination, Third World AIDS education programmes use local popular culture to strengthen rather than weaken collective community values and self-esteem.[5] In the meantime the bitter irony remains that as Western commentators retreat behind the defensive stockades of racism and homophobia, they shut their ears and eyes to those who have developed effective preventive measures against the further transmission of HIV.

Dr Allan Brandt has argued forcefully that, "there will be no simple answer to this health crisis."[6] He points out that no health promotion campaign based on fear has ever proved effective, and that no single intervention, not even a vaccine, "will adequately address the complexities of the AIDS epidemic." The Director of the World Health Organization's AIDS Programme has emphasized that: "We are still in the early phases of a global epidemic whose first decade gives every reason for concern about the future of global AIDS . . . There is no public health rationale to justify isolation, quarantine, or other discriminatory measures based solely on a person's HIV infection status . . . Discrimination will undermine the entire national information and education programme: thus discrimination itself can endanger public health." By taking refuge in the most vicious resurgence of racist and homophobic victim-blaming, the West runs the dreadful risk now of encouraging the *increased* incidence of HIV amongst heterosexuals because it is unable to question its own stupefying legacy of sexual and racial prejudice, ignorance, and fear. In the face of such widespread, murderous folly, we can only affirm the value and dignity of human life in all its diversity. As James Baldwin has observed: "each of us is unique, irreplaceable, and passing through. But, it seems to me that it is precisely our irreplaceability, uniqueness, mortality, that is the splendour of the human connection. That isolation and death are certain and universal clarifies our responsibility."[8]

Notes

Parts of this article were originally written as a leaflet for British journalists, commissioned by the UK Non-Government Organization (NGO) AIDS Consortium for the Third World.

1. Cindy Patton, "Inventing African Aids", *City Limits*, issue 363, 15–22 September 1988, p. 85.

2. Sander L. Gilman, *Disease and Representation: Images of Illness from Madness to Aids*, London 1988, p. 1.

3. Simon Watney, "Missionary Politics: Aids, Africa and Race", *Differences: A Feminist Journal of Cultural Studies* vol. 1, no. 1, Indiana 1988.

4. Renée Sabatier, *Blaming Others: Prejudice, Race and Worldwide AIDS*, London 1988, p. 92.

5. Ibid., p. 92.

6. Allan M. Brandt, "Aids in Historical Perspective: Four Lessons from the History of Sexually Transmitted Diseases", *American Journal of Public Health*, vol. 78, no. 4, April 1988, p. 28.

7. Jonathan Mann, "Opening Statement to the World Summit of Ministers of Health", London, 26 January 1988. Reported in *The Guardian*, 27 January 1988, p. 2.

8. James Baldwin, *The Evidence of Things Not Seen*, New York 1985, p. 52.

KEITH ALCORN

AIDS IN THE PUBLIC SPHERE

How a Broadcasting System in Crisis Dealt With an Epidemic

Since 1985 I have been talking to people about AIDS and safer sex, first at London Lesbian and Gay Switchboard, and since December 1986, at the National AIDS Helpline.

During that time I have observed the reporting of the epidemic closely, and seen the ebb and flow of a public "crisis" which transcends the category of moral panic. I have also become acutely aware of the extent to which a public debate over AIDS was constructed by the institutional imperatives of broadcasting, most notably in the AIDS Television Week in March 1987. This was a week of programmes about AIDS, and television companies co-ordinated their schedules to ensure the widest possible audience for the subject.

These institutional imperatives, shared by all the networks, can be mapped in three ways. The first is the economic terrain, to which I will return in my conclusion. For now, it is necessary to point out the importance of media markets, both in newspapers and television. Much public knowledge about AIDS was produced under the specific conditions and pressures of the UK tabloid market. AIDS appeared during a period of vigorous ideological conflict in the UK, and a large part of that struggle took place in the pages of the popular press.

This was also a period of global restructuring of the media economy. The British outlets of News International, for instance, now play a crucial part in the global designs of Rupert Murdoch, providing the cash to pay interest on huge loans taken out to buy US TV stations.[1] The effect this has on British television is the creation of a situation of perpetual uneasiness, exacerbated by the government's hostility towards the present structure of British broadcasting, and by a technology/profit-led trend towards the globalization and liberalization of all broadcasting systems.

The second is the terrain of public accountability, or politics in the more traditional sense. As this volume emphasizes, the response of the British government to the epidemic was highly negligent, yet it mirrored television's conception of its audience, with its reference to "the general population". Television executives were asked to use their power to make up for the shortcomings of the government AIDS campaign, which had been widely criticized as too little and too late. I will discuss these negotiations between the broadcasters and the Department of Health and Social Security (DHSS) below, but for now it is important to emphasize the absence of AIDS from the political agenda of television. *Weekend World* was the only "political" programme to pay attention to the politics of AIDS during AIDS Television Week, which stuck rigidly to the agenda of a public debate initiated by the press and the priorities of the "general population".

The third imperative emerges as one of containment. Television as an institution contains and accommodates the many anxieties and disturbances created by AIDS. This is not merely a question of welfarism, but also of psychic imperatives, and we should look to Simon Watney's *Policing Desire* and Leo Bersani's essay "Is The Rectum A Grave" for some powerful suggestions about the way in which:

> . . . consent for social policy is grafted from desire itself, as political prescriptions are understood to protect heterosexual identities.

Time and again, threats to heterosexuality and the private space of the home, in the form of sex education about "deviants", homosexuality on television and family members who turn out to be gay ("Goodbye Sailor — I'm divorcing gay sailor," says Gillian[2]), produce the homosexual as:

> . . . a regulatory and admonitory sign which has come to occupy a most peculiar and centrally privileged position in the government of the home.[3]

The Britishness of Television Week:
Broadcasting institutions found themselves with a number of conflicting demands in their response to AIDS, conflicts which are clearly signposted in much of the broadcast material, and particularly *Day to Day : The AIDS Debate* which is analysed below.

The tension lies in the notion of public service broadcasting. The common thread running through AIDS Television Week was the need to balance education as part of a public health campaign with the institutional needs of television, particularly the maintenance of a tradition of "objective", independent programme-making, with its conventions of balance.

AIDS Television Week and the Government health education campaign have been widely seen as examples to the world. No other West European countries have attacked the subject with such intensity, either because health education initiatives began much earlier, as in Holland and Scandinavia, or because constraints of social custom and media structure have prevented such concerted action, as in France and Italy. Although the need for a Europe-wide strategy on research and treatment has been agreed, the national limits of health education strategies are rigorously observed.

The British response is local and specific partly because of the structure of broadcasting in the United Kingdom, which is itself connected with notions of national identity, but also because of the pattern of emergence of HIV in the UK.

In each country affected by HIV the pattern of its emergence has been related to national-historical characteristics which are reflected in broadcasting structures. In France and Belgium, a large proportion of those with HIV are Africans; in Spain and Italy there is a prevalence of HIV among drug injectors. Without engaging in a detailed contrast, it should be noted that the social formations that have produced the Mediterranean pattern of AIDS reflect the historical under-development of these regions in relation to Northern Europe and America.[4] AIDS is thus deeply embedded in the social formation, and cannot be understood as a public issue without reference to the formation of the public sphere in which it appears.

In the UK, broadcasting was expected to respond at the point when the virus threatened to "leak" into "the general population". The prior indifference of British broadcasters to AIDS — in terms of health education rather than curiosity or crisis — is all the more shocking when one considers the claims of broadcasting institutions, particularly the BBC, to be caring institutions.[5]

Broadcasting in the United Kingdom has developed primarily as a national cultural institution which regularly uses the monarchy to organize and validate its activities. It has also risen to the occasion of several national crises that have further enhanced its authority. Scannell argues that after the General Strike of 1926 the BBC was increasingly drawn into the corporate apparatus of government, and persuaded to downplay social and diplomatic tensions during the 1930s. Subsequently the BBC has been careful to hold to a more critical notion of the public interest, one in which broadcasters have the right to investigate and challenge state policy while enjoying the paradoxical advantage of a state monopoly to hold their audience.[6]

A comparison of Television Week with wartime broadcasting would be facile, but it was nevertheless an unprecedented peacetime event. Although broadcasters have often covered events of national importance on separate channels, it was the first occasion when networks co-operated in their scheduling. Apart from the Apollo moon landings, Television Week was probably the first event not concerned with the monarchy, sport or parliamentary politics to dominate the schedules. Television Week was thus an unprecedented event, not only in terms of co-operation between broadcasters, but also in terms of scale.

The original suggestion, following discussions between the networks instigated by Sir Kenneth Stowe, permanent secretary at the DHSS, had been for a single programme broadcast simultaneously across four channels. The DHSS had suggested that broadcasters might have something to contribute to its AIDS information campaign nearly eight months after it had launched a newspaper advertising campaign, criticized by the press, public and voluntary organizations as vague and confusing.

By November 1986 however, the campaign was moving into higher gear. It was designed to develop in four phases — national newspaper adverts, billboard advertising, a youth campaign and a leaflet drop to every home in the country, using the slogan "AIDS —Don't die of ignorance." Television advertising on both BBC and ITV was to follow in the early months of 1987.

It was expected that this campaign would lead to a massive increase in public awareness of AIDS, but having stimulated public awareness, would it satisfy the demand for information? It was felt within the DHSS that television had a part to play not only in reaching the widest audience, but also in providing more accessible information.

Thus on 19 November 1986, officials of the DHSS, including the Chief Medical Officer, Sir Donald Acheson, BBC executives and an official of the Cabinet Office met to discuss the need for the widest possible public health campaign. It was felt that such a campaign should stress three messages: "Cut down on partners; Use condoms if you are not sure about your partners; Do not share needles if you must persist in injecting drugs."

By 15 December discussion and planning within the BBC was advanced enough for an internal meeting to conclude that the original suggestion of a four channel "simulcast" would "produce party political irritation". There was concern throughout the preparation of Television Week that such a revolution in scheduling practices would set a precedent which could be repeated in more contentious circumstances. It was also felt that, as public awareness increased, such a move might be unnecessary. A two channel broadcast was approved, *AIDS — The Facts*, presented by Janice Long and Ian Dury.

It was also emphasized that the BBC had no licence to preach, yet there was little discussion of the "moral" aspect during the planning of Television Week. At the beginning of a campaign which was significantly to extend the boundaries of public discussion about sex, television executives spent very little time discussing the possible storm over the corruption of public morals, according to documents I have seen.

Mick Rhodes, head of science features, originally suggested that any simulcast should cover three areas: "How do you catch AIDS? How do you avoid catching it? If you catch it, what do you do?" By 12 January the IBA had ruled out any prospect of a long simulcast, but accepted the principle of a short programme. It was decided that the Television Week would take place at the end of February, after a short lull in the government advertising campaign. Three days later, representatives of the BBC, ITV and the DHSS met to discuss the campaign once again, and it was noted that the Secretary of State for the DHSS, Norman Fowler, would be visiting the United States at the end of January. His visit was to receive extensive news coverage as an integral part of both the government and the television public health campaigns.

In the meantime, BBC Radio 1 had already launched its own public health campaign, derived from its experience with *Drug Alert*, a week of programming backed up with a telephone helpline that had been highly successful in 1985 and 1986. It was realized during this campaign that a large proportion of the callers to the *Drug Alert* helpline needed information about AIDS, and Radio 1, with an audience of 19 million each week, of whom 70 per cent are in the 16–34 age group, was clearly an effective way of reaching the age group said to be most at risk from AIDS.

The Radio 1 Play Safe campaign began on 14 December 1986, with a 48-minute documentary which stressed that listeners should limit their number of partners and use condoms, and emphasized that they could call the National Advisory Service on AIDS for more information, including a free information pack. This contained several leaflets reiterating basic "facts" about AIDS, and a letter from the then Director General of the BBC, Sir Alisdair Milne, designed to allay parents' fears about the explicit contents of the information pack!

In contrast, one highly significant feature of Television Week was the disavowal of moral responses to the epidemic, despite the keenness of some Thatcherites for a return to the primacy of the family, the keystone of Mrs Thatcher's ideological world view.[7] Television Week did force a frank discussion of sexuality, although the taboo on representations of sexuality remained in force.

Since the first major clash between gays and the moral right in the *Gay News* blasphemy trial, there has been a mindfulness that the full force of the law is available to restrict and crush any representations of lesbian and gay life. Similarly concern about pornography and obscenity in broadcasting has escalated in a series of "moral panics" that have expanded the scope of regulation in the private sphere after a period of relaxation.

Television executives were thus acutely aware by late 1986 that they were under severe pressure to cooperate with the government in enforcing standards of decency and morality. A revision of the Obscene Publications Act to cover television was planned, and despite the failure of the Churchill amendment to that Act, Conservative opinion supported greater restriction on the content of television even as the deregulation of cultural markets was taking place. The one coherent strand running through Conservative communications policy has been reactive measures to protect "public morals" and "national security". From the licencing of cable television to the acceptance of satellite and the floating of the idea of subscription television, there has been a more consistent emphasis on the control of indecency than on the deregulation of broadcasting.

The threat of the Churchill amendment had in itself been successful in censoring television, but it had not eradicated images of homosexuality from the screen. During 1986 the BBC's largest audience programme, *Eastenders*, introduced two gay characters living in a "pretended family relationship", while Channel 4's *Brookside* dealt with the coming-out of a young gay man to his family. These portrayals within a specialized genre of television could not redress the general absence of gays from television, nor could they disguise the discomfort of adults talking about sex in their own homes. The central institutional problem of Television Week involved talking about sex for viewing at home. Television Week undermined television's conception of its audience by threatening to disrupt the delicate balance between consumerism and family values that informs it. The family, "the miserably impoverished core of television's understanding of its actual audience," has been a crucial term in the discourse of public service broadcasting, structuring schedules, modes of address and content.[8] It has also served to enhance the reputation and authority of British broadcasting by constantly reiterating a triangular relationship between royal family, viewing family and national family through an obsessive coverage of royalty, marriage, divorce, babies and home-making, emphasizing family experience as its common currency. This coverage has an essentially didactic character, not only in terms of its relentless heterosexism, but also in the task it performs of stabilizing national identity through an alignment with a past symbolized by the royal family and the national heritage.[9]

At the same time, however, television often addresses us as consumers with desires that cut against the logic of family values, particularly through the use of sexuality in advertising. Television Week threatened to explode the limited repertoire of sexual life-styles on offer by revealing how un-monogamous, un-heterosexual and "unusual" the everyday sexuality of the British really is.

Day to Day: The AIDS Debate
One programme broadcast during Television Week provides considerable insight into AIDS in the "public sphere".

The AIDS Debate, a special edition of the BBC 1 programme *Day to Day*, was broadcast between 10.30 and 11.50 pm on Friday, 27 February 1987 on BBC 1. It attracted an estimated audience of 4.5 million, of whom at least one third were over fifty-five.

Quite apart from the range of opinions expressed, *The AIDS Debate* is interesting because of its institutional context. *Day to Day*, has a borrowed format, originated by the *Oprah Winfrey Show* in the United States, and deals with a mixture of serious and trivial issues, always constituted as social problems which require a cooperative solution. The studio audience is usually recruited by a television trailer advertising the theme of the show, soliciting people with opinions on the subject. It is thus a self-selecting audience, but nevertheless an audience thoroughly researched by the producers and policed by presenter Robert Kilroy-Silk, a former "moderate" Labour MP.

At the time of broadcast *Day to Day* was a new show, part of the BBC's new daytime schedules. It thus represented an attempt to come to terms with the new and more competitive structure of British television forced on the BBC by the emergence of commercial breakfast television (which opened the door to round the clock television), and government reluctance to subsidize the BBC through the licence fee (which encouraged a greater emphasis on audience ratings in order to justify the continued high level of that fee). The BBC was required to develop formats of programming across the schedules which could draw larger audiences.

The AIDS Debate was shifted to the late evening slot partly to attract a larger audience, but also to attract a different audience —the people most likely to be at risk from AIDS. This seems a naïve programming strategy, since Friday night is a time many younger people choose to socialize rather than watch television, and there is evidence that this first wave of programmes did not reach young people. *The AIDS Debate* did reach their parents however; 65 per cent of the audience was estimated to be over thirty-five, and according to a *BARB* poll, the presenter was appreciated more by over thirty-fives than the young. Similarly, the over thirty-fives were more likely to agree that the participants were well chosen and the debate easy to follow. The programme received an Appreciation Index of 79, compared with 80 for *AIDS—The Facts*, and 83 for *QED:AIDS*, and from information supplied it is clear that in the broadcasters' terms, there was a very high appreciation ot *The AIDS Debate*, as one of the most factual programmes in Television Week.[10]

If *The AIDS Debate* was appreciated, however, it was because its format was recognizable. Throughout Television Week, AIDS was negotiated within the conventional formats of television. In the following section, I want to look more closely at how conflicts over the meaning of AIDS were contained, organized and articulated within the existing framework of television broadcasting.

Symptoms of a Killer Disease

The most common event in Television Week was the interview. One was particularly important, an interview which opened *The AIDS Debate*. It was with Terry Madeley, a British man with AIDS, who appeared to be fairly well and not at all apologetic for his condition. Terry was one of the pivotal figures of *The AIDS Debate*, his status fluctuating between that of a mere symptom and a responsible PWA. His was the face the camera constantly sought out for reaction shots.

Television documentaries and current affairs programmes often use a personal story to introduce debates and issues. Their justification is invariably identification, which "operates in two modes — the transitive sense of identifying self in relation to the difference of the other, and the reflexive sense of identifying self in a relation of resemblance to the other."[11] This seems a particularly pertinent observation in the light of Terry Madeley, a gay man with AIDS, and in terms of the function he performs within *The AIDS Debate*.

There seem to be two questions posed to the viewer in the presentation of this interviewee: "Do you want to end up like this?" and "What shall we do about people like him?" These questions run through the programme, motivating a high degree of information-giving and warning, and questions about attitudes towards PWA's.

Terry's sickness is authenticated by his account of "a pleasant daily function turned into feeling as though you've got a graze as long as Blackpool seafront" — the effect of internal herpes. This account of symptoms seems at once to invite identification, pulling against the difference inscribed in Terry's homosexuality, and yet to produce Terry over and over again as a symptom, a person whose identity is circumscribed by his diagnosis.

Information about AIDS is produced in a personal context here, in deference to the structural demands of the programme. The audience has probably learnt more about living with AIDS in the past few minutes than they've ever done before, and now have the opportunity to ask themselves, "How would I deal with it if this was me or my family?" or "How do I think this problem should be dealt with?" At this point we have to note that Terry is emblematic of representations of gay men with AIDS as white, middle-class, fairly camp and funny.

The audience is being offered shifting positions of identification throughout *The AIDS Debate* — people at risk, citizens responding to a government campaign, people without AIDS. *The AIDS Debate* is regularly interrupted by opinion polls and by phone-in sections which comment on the three questions asked at the beginning and on the matters under discussion in the studio. They appear to provide a degree of accountability to the programme itself, but give participants no influence, and should be seen as autonomous segments which are used within the format to enhance notions of broad debate and greater public awareness. They have an inclusive appearance, but seem to function merely as "story space" or a separate programme/story going on within the discourse of *The AIDS Debate*, and indeed are signposted as a link-up with the *Open Air* programme, signalling the special status of the topic under discussion.[12] Yet while they don't affect the direction of the debate, they do produce the surprising evidence that a large number of callers want more information about AIDS and appear to be using the *Open Air* phone-in as an advice service, a totally unintended outcome!

These two devices set an agenda which is partially undermined by the demand for more information about AIDS. This demand could be ascribed to the fact that the AIDS campaign had only begun that night, but equally, it could be argued that it was an unequivocal reply to the question, "Have the Government got the AIDS campaign right?"

The effectiveness of the campaign is significantly the first item on the agenda. This in itself is a radical departure from usual broadcasting practice; it proposes a public sphere in which official statements can be held accountable, not merely through the agency of the interviewer but through a direct audience reaction. At this point it is important to note that a traditional political discourse has been efficiently erased from *The AIDS Debate*. There are no party representatives to comment on the public health campaign, unlike

Weekend World earlier in the year, which had invited party health representatives to debate the campaign. This absence is unusual and significant given the parliamentary traditions inscribed in current affairs broadcasting, and an ironic omission in view of the public service tradition invoked in Television Week. The practice of balance relies instead on views from other social constituencies to provide an "objective" discussion: constituencies in civil society such as gays, feminists, youth, voluntary agencies and the moral right.

Accountability is an increasingly important and explicit part of television discourse. To some extent this is a response to attacks on the medium from both politicians and viewers who have alleged unaccountability. It is thus a strategy to enhance notions of public service broadcasting, which might explain why *Day to Day, Open Air* and *Question Time* are all BBC productions (although it should be noted that Channel Four's *Right To Reply* was the precursor of *Open Air*). It is also a strategy which increases the interpretation of the public and private worlds through television, and which blurs the modes of address and breaks down the barriers between media institutions and their publics. For instance, viewers are invited to "put their views to" public figures "here to answer your questions". Television increasingly uses reportage of comment in the form of letters and phone-ins to create effects of intimacy, immediacy and accountability.

Yet accountability also involves a problem of balancing the demands of delivering a service without genuine market conditions, creating ways of making broadcasting more responsive to its market and yet remaining accountable to autonomous professional standards. *The AIDS Debate* is thus trying to juggle several different problems of accountability: the need for politicians to use television to legitimate political decisions; the need for broadcasters to investigate public issues according to their own standards and the need for broadcasters to test the public response to a campaign that would be impossible without broadcasters' co-operation.

Real People and Unrealistic Measures

The AIDS Debate tried to deal with questions about drugs, morality, antibody testing and punitive measures against PWA's. The debate was largely confined to personal issues until the subject of compulsory testing was brought up, via the presentation of an opinion poll, interchangeable with many others that have appeared in the *Sun*, the *News of the World* or the *People*, which concluded that a majority of respondents supported the compulsory identification of seropositives.

The case for compulsory testing is put by Christopher Monckton, at the time deputy editor of *Today* newspaper and formerly an editor of the *Universe*, the Catholic newspaper owned in part by his family. Monckton has also been a member of Mrs Thatcher's Policy Unit, and his grasp of Thatcherite rhetoric is demonstrated in his appeal, over-riding the actual studio audience, to the "real people" at home, and in his use of the Thatcherite "you", echoed by Graham Webster-Gardiner of the Conservative Family Campaign later in the debate.

Monckton's invocation of the "real people" is an attempt to shift the agenda through an attack on the way the programme has organized its agenda in advance, "a carefully selected audience" being a staple of television talk shows. It is also an attack on the right of various representative participants to speak —politicians for the government and doctors for the medical profession, and an attack on gay men, who, since they are not part of the "general population", cannot be "real people". Monckton is speaking to an audience of his own choice, one which apportions people to "risk groups" rather than allowing people to change their behaviour. This has the effect of disrupting the identifications offered in earlier discussions about behaviour changes, and returns victim-blaming and punitive measures to the agenda.

Kilroy is quick to jump to the defence of the studio audience, since this is a direct attack on his own credibility as presenter. Having heard the proposal for compulsory testing, Kilroy asks Dr Michael Adler to reply first. Adler chooses not to explain why a programme of mass testing is impracticable, unreliable and immensely expensive, but instead discusses testing in terms of rights. There is a remarkable absence throughout this programme segment of any coherent argument against compulsory testing, which is not, as Dr Adler claims, a complex question. No one gets the opportunity to explain that it doesn't work until Dr Ray Brettle attempts to intervene, but Kilroy suppresses a fuller explanation shortly afterwards in order to bring in a more extreme voice than Monckton, who, although he isn't named, I recognize to be Graham

Webster-Gardiner, chairman of the Conservative Family Campaign, whose line is "lock them up."

At this point, Kilroy suddenly begins to take sides. Rather than using Dr Adler to oppose this argument, he questions Gardiner himself, drawing on the positions which Adler has just staked out, invoking images of internment and concentration camps. His appeal here is to the liberal imagination, in which the camps are the index of inhumanity and intolerance, and Gardiner, with his advocacy of internment, can be seen to be pushing against the outer limits of liberal democracy. Thus Kilroy reinforces the liberal, co-operative, consensus-seeking objectives of *The AIDS Debate*, before handing over to Terry Madeley, who ties together notions of real people and unrealistic measures in a question to everyone about personal responsibility which efficiently returns choice rather than coercion to the top of the agenda. Terry is used here as a "real person with AIDS", reminding us that although in the terms of television's discourse, "real people" can only ever be symptoms or witnesses of the problem under discussion, they cannot always be controlled by the presenter or the format.

Jonathan Grimshaw of Body Positive is then invited to speak, as a person with HIV. While what he says is in itself quite coherent, it still doesn't defuse the potent notion that mass testing is a solution, and Monckton is quick to point out that condoms too are a less than perfect solution to the "spread of AIDS". But is isolation a solution? Monckton denies that it is on his agenda, but discussion of the topic leads to the clearest contrast between libertarian and authoritarian positions, as a woman replies to Michal Adler's appeal for faith in voluntary behaviour changes with a call for positive steps to test and quarantine people.

It is left to Norman Fowler, addressed as Minister in this instance to underline his authority, to reject the call for compulsory testing. In this segment the abstract debate over public policy has been punctured just once, by Terry Madeley, and it is the freedom given him to make his intervention which seems to me the most important indicator of the consensus which the show hopes to promote, a consensus in which "compassion" and "human rights" are more important than coercion. These are institutional demands which can be equated with freedom of speech, jealously protected by television, and they reflect the extent to which broadcasters seek to ground *The AIDS Debate* in the ethics of public service broadcasting

— compassionate, Christian and socially cohesive. The drive towards a consensual and ethically correct solution in the more controversial editions of *Kilroy* I have watched recently, most notably in a heated confrontation over apartheid broadcast during the week ending 22 April 1988, is strongly marked. I find the concluding sequence of *The AIDS Debate* particularly memorable; after an interview with Terry Madeley's mother, a strikingly cheery woman who epitomized the Loving Mum, Terry is asked what he thought of his Mums's words. "I think you should put my Mum on the National Health!" he replies.

The After-life of Television Week: *Remember Terry* and *The Visit*
If Television Week marked the first serious attempt by British television to deal with the epidemic, it was also important because it set the tone of future coverage of HIV-related issues. Television producers at once became aware of the potential audience for programmes about AIDS, and since March 1987 almost every genre of television, from drama (*Intimate Contact* and *Sweet As You Are*) through current affairs to documentary (*Remember Terry* and *The Visit*) has sought to remove AIDS from the stranglehold of science programming and present the personal and human dimensions of the epidemic. The most ambitious attempt was a six part series entitled *AIDS Now* commissioned by Channel Four and shown in the first months of 1988. The series included reports on AIDS in Africa and the likelihood of a heterosexual epidemic, and covered these topics with traditional documentary voyeurism — prostitutes shot from car windows, a map showing the journeys of HIV-positive drug injectors in the UK, and a presentation of Africa that dwelt unrelentingly on the dehumanization of "AIDS victims" and hardly acknowledged the economic and cultural imperialism that has constructed the epidemic in central Africa.

Documentary programmes produced for the BBC have generally been more innovative and sensitive than the shabby sensationalism of *AIDS Now*, but have been unable to avoid reproducing people with AIDS as victims. The programmes analysed below are two of the many personal stories that have attempted to address sympathetically the many "risk groups" or audiences of television's public.

Remember Terry was a one-hour documentary broadcast in November 1987 on BBC 2 at 8 pm. It was made by Patty Coldwell of BBC Manchester and was described as, "a personal tribute to the first man to come out with AIDS on British television." We should note the signposting of the extraordinary in this description, which is a common identifying feature of television coverage of the subject. Yet *Remember Terry* is in some ways a deeply ordinary piece of television, unlike much of the output during Television Week itself. It is a representation of a gay man who could be criticized as stereotypical, the conventional drama queen permitted to appear on TV. It is organized in the usual style of verité documentary as a realistic narrative in which we ignore the fact that Patty's arrival in the hospital room must be staged, like so many other moments of "naturalness". It is ordinary in the sense that it follows a character who is clearly signalled as extraordinary, as television documentaries do.

It *is* exceptional in the way that it foregrounds the bonds of friendship between producer and subject, implying that it is in no way unusual for television to jettison its subjects after filming. It questions the role of the reporter as an objective viewer, since Patty Coldwell is involved quite deeply in the action; when Terry finally dies, she helps orchestrate the funeral.

The "ordinary/extraordinary" distinction seems a useful frame in which to analyse this piece of television, since it weaves themes of celebrity and morbidity which, although not parts of everyday life, are constant themes of television discourse.

Terry Madeley is introduced by a clip from *Day to Day*, which established him as a personable advocate for the rights and experiences of PWA's, and we follow him to *Open Air Special*, and the pinnacle of celebrity, *Wogan*, as he becomes a new form of media personality, the telegenic PWA.

Much television coverage of AIDS has been preoccupied with morbidity and with transforming the complex symptoms of AIDS into a recognizable image. These images cannot by any stretch of the liberal imagination be called telegenic, yet they are what AIDS looks like, as Simon Watney argues in "The Subject of AIDS".[13]

Remember Terry attempts to exhibit the normal and ordinary conditions in which a PWA exists, both material and psychic, and succeeds in conveying a great deal of information. It exposes the uncertainty that follows an HIV positive diagnosis, the constant stress of hospitalization, drugs and remission in a way that no previous programme has done, and also raises issues about confidentiality, care partners, grieving and confronting death that are equally stressful for PWA's.

It does this however, within another discourse, the discourse of televized homosexuality. Representation of the subject is always already structured in advance by the broadcasting institution through time-slot, assumed audience and format (current affairs, drama, comedy), and lesbians and gays have emerged to "speak for themselves" only since the advent of minority programming. Instances in which lesbians and gays have had editorial control of British TV programmes in which they are represented are few.

Thus it is perfectly ordinary for Patty Coldwell to ask, on behalf of the assumed audience, "Why is Terry gay?" as if this was an extraordinary fact that requires explanation; and to proceed with a highly conventional explanation, that it was because he grew up almost exclusively among women.

The Visit was an 80-minute documentary in a series presented by Desmond Wilcox, who had been dispatched to San Francisco in order to introduce the experience of living with AIDS to a hetero-sexual audience in the UK. *The Visit* might more accurately be called *The Intrusion*; various scenarios of the hardship and heroism of US PWA's have been served up to British audiences, and Wilcox's visit to AIDS educator Richard Rector is, however well-meaning, still an attempt to mediate the experience of AIDS for a television audience assumed to be unfamiliar with the culture that has emerged in San Francisco.

For Richard Rector, educating people about *living* with AIDS is the priority; yet *The Visit* can only comprehend this within a frame that emphasizes the imminent death not only of the star of the show but thousands of others who are condemned as pleasure-seekers and libertines by a visual shorthand which consistently uses a disco to signify gay men.

The Visit is necessarily read with reference to other visits that preceded it, those of tabloid reporters or Norman Fowler, who as Secretary of State visited "The AIDS capital of North America" before Television Week. Such visits emphasized the scale of the human disaster in San Francisco without permitting any message about the overwhelming success of the gay community in promoting Safer Sex and creating a health-care programme that reflects the needs of the communities affected. For Wilcox, the task was to redress this information gap.

Yet *The Visit* dwells quite persistently on death, despite the best efforts of Richard Rector, who is quite painfully aware of his dependence on the television crew and producer for any opportunity to educate people about living with AIDS. Once again we see a documentary subject pinioned by the presenter into dredging up the most painful memories and experiences to serve the mechanism of identification upon which all good television is presumed to operate.

The Visit is at times a remarkable tribute to the people who are fighting the epidemic and living with AIDS, but we should beware the apparent neutrality or even sympathy of any television documentary. We've been aware for nearly fifteen years of the tyranny of naturalism in television, and many of the points I have noted could equally well be applied to any other documentary subject. Television has been remarkably keen to cover AIDS, precisely because it is unfamiliar and simultaneously offers the opportunity for new styles of coverage and a personalization of the epidemic that tends to undermine any critical analysis of the problems producers face in bringing the subject into the home.

Conclusion

AIDS became a special kind of public emergency in Britain during the 1980s because of the intervention of the mass media and the inaction of the government. It was correctly seen as a social crisis, but public understanding of why this was so remained vague, and public debate polarized around two abstractions: "morality", and controlling "the spread of AIDS". Throughout this debate only gays and blacks challenged the ways in which knowledge about AIDS was being produced and framed. In the political conditions of eighties Britain such marginal voices took nearly five years to penetrate the schedules of television, and they have still not done so in the United States, a nation where more than a million people are already infected with HIV.

Television Week was a unique attempt to deal with that public emergency in the face of the coyness of early government campaigns. Its key features were co-operation between television channels; an attempt to talk frankly about sex while negotiating the problem of "taste and decency" which in itself had made AIDS an uncomfortable subject; an attempt to promote an ethos of compassion and tolerance towards PWA's in the public service tradition that is the hallmark of the BBC; an attempt to provide a coherent and unified body of information about AIDS in line with DHSS guidelines, and finally, a tendency to amplify the event as a news and current affairs story in itself.

The Television Week was also an attempt to influence the public debate over AIDS by using the "objective" journalistic authority of broadcasting to reiterate the danger of a heterosexual epidemic, and to convey more detailed information about AIDS than the government campaign had done.

The AIDS Debate largely suppressed the question of government complicity in the epidemic, just as it suppressed questions of morality. A strong refusal to make any moral judgements has marked the British AIDS campaign, in strong contrast to the moral content of federal AIDS education in the USA. This refusal has been based on a mistaken compromise statement — stick to one partner — which serves to pacify religious critics. Sticking to one partner is clearly murderous advice if that partner is unknowingly infected, and another refusal, to admit the possible scale of infection that already exists, has further influenced policy in the UK towards this mistaken compromise.

The rhetoric of the government's campaign has nevertheless produced a moral agenda in which "promiscuity" is once again agreed to be socially dangerous, and in which the "general population" is seen to exclude gays and drug users. Gay men have never been the subject of direct address by a government campaign, thus emphasizing their marginalization and their invisibility in society.

If the essential ideological thrust of neo-liberalism is to re-establish the market as the *only* public sphere, the future funding of AIDS related broadcasting is likely to be dictated by news values, commercial interests, public emergency and private philanthropy.

Rather than accepting that future access to producing public representations of AIDS should be through private funding, workers in AIDS should work actively with education departments in all television companies to negotiate a long-term strategy in which the public service tradition and the back-up services available together use television for the purposes of health education.

This is a strategy which would begin to uncouple broadcasting from its embrace with state institutions like the DHSS and claim public service broadcasting for self-defined publics. The danger in this strategy is that public service broadcasting will become identified with special interest groups unless we accept that notions of balance and objectivity in television are going to have to be radically de-centred, in a politicization of television akin to that in Holland, which, relies on a pluralist notion of rights and democracy throughout society.[14]

Within the next few years television in the UK faces a serious disruption signalled by the November 1988 White Paper on Broadcasting. The White Paper contains proposals not only to open a new, regionally based television channel, but also to alter the delicately balanced funding arrangements of British television.

It is intended that the BBC should gradually become a subscription based service, that the franchises of the regional independent companies should be auctioned to the highest bidder, and that there should be a greater degree of competition in the television advertising market. Satellite and cable television will also gain larger audience shares.

These proposals may lead to a lowering of quality, since the new arrangements will largely emphasize the pursuit of mass audiences within a highly fragmented market, making an event like Television Week impossible and signalling the decline of programme-making which would treat AIDS seriously and sympathetically.

One of the chief dangers of the new arrangements is a further "tabloidization" of television, with an increased reliance on devices like the celebrity, the opinion poll, and the "true confession" to draw audiences, as *First AIDS* illustrated. One ITV executive later remarked that he saw in *First AIDS* a model for future current affairs broadcasting. In such circumstances it seems essential to maintain a critical adherence to the notion of public service broadcasting, which should not be abandoned despite its past inflexibility over questions of gender, race, sexuality and regionalism. In order to maintain a debate over AIDS in the public sphere we need to maintain that public sphere even as we challenge the dominant practices of televisual representation.

Notes

I would like to thank David Cardiff of the Polytechnic of Central London and Simon Watney for their comments on previous versions of these arguments, and Keith Smith of Broadcasting Support Services for allowing me access to documents pertaining to AIDS Television Week.

1. Douglas Gomery, "Vertical Integration, Horizontal Regulation; The Growth of Rupert Murdoch's US Media Empire", *Screen*, vol. 27, no. 3/4.
2. *The Star*, 3 July 1986.
3. Simon Watney, "The Spectacle of AIDS", *October*, no. 42, 1988.
4. Alan Lipietz, *Mirages and Miracles: The Crisis of Global Fordism*, London 1987, pp. 113–30.
5. In a speech to the 1987 Social Action Broadcasting conference, Geraint Stanley Jones described the BBC as "expected to care", and outlined the history of social and moral concern which underlies the public service tradition. To imply that this lies in a unified tradition of welfarism is however to ignore the complex motives behind welfarism, as Lee and Raban show in "Welfare and Ideology", in *Social Policy and Social Welfare* (ed. M. Loney, D. Boswell, and J. Clarke), London 1983.
6. Paddy Scannell, "Conspiracy of Silence", in *State and Society in Contemporary Britain* (ed. G. McLennan), London 1986.
7. Alan O'Shea, "Trusting the People", in *Formations of Nation and People*, London 1984.
8. Simon Watney, *Policing Desire: Pornography, AIDS and the Media*, London 1987, p. 121; see also pp. 98–100.
9. Patrick Wright, *On Living in an Old Country*, London 1986, pp. 135–61.
10. "Public Attitudes to AIDS", BBC Internal Research Document, April 1987.
11. Simon Watney, "The Spectacle of AIDS", op. cit.
12. Margaret Morse, "Talk, Talk, Talk: The Space of Discourse in Television", *Screen*, vol. 26, no. 2, 1985.
13. Simon Watney, "The Subject of AIDS", *Copyright*, vol. 1, no. 1, reprinted in P. Aggleton et al (eds.), *AIDS: Social Representations, Social Practices*, London 1989.
14. Kees Brants, "Broadcasting and Politics in the Netherlands", in *Broadcasting and Politics in Western Europe* (ed. Raymond Kuhn), London 1985.

JONATHAN GRIMSHAW

THE INDIVIDUAL CHALLENGE

Last night, as expected, I had a telephone call from someone I have met only once but who has phoned me once a week for the past two years. This person wants, desperately, to live. He rings me for advice and for reassurance that all the things he is doing to protect his health — to try to stay alive — are the right things. Like me, he has HIV-1.

Like me, he had seen the *Nine O'Clock News* last night and heard a report that 90 per cent, perhaps more, of people with HIV will develop AIDS within ten years. We discussed this and then, just before putting the phone down, he said, "It's a bit much isn't it, you try so hard to stay alive and then they keep telling you you're going to die," and I agreed that yes, it was a bit much.

I am sure that Drs Sir Donald Acheson (the Chief Medical Officer) and Spencer Hagard (Director of the Health Education Authority) would, if they had to care for people with HIV as their patients, follow good counselling procedure and advise those patients to do everything they could to protect their immune systems: avoid stress, eat a balanced diet, get plenty of rest, avoid sexually transmitted diseases, change to a healthier lifestyle.

I wonder what Sir Donald or Spencer would say to me if I was their patient and, in response to their advice I retorted, "What is the point of my doing any of these things? Why should I re-arrange my life and my priorities in an effort to stay well when I saw you on television last night as good as saying that I'd have AIDS within ten years ... AIDS is fatal isn't it? You give me no hope because what you're really saying is that nothing I do will make any difference."

My telephone friend's doctor has not told him that AIDS would be virtually inevitable; that doctor is going to be in some difficulty when my friend attends for his next appointment.

The Health Education Authority (HEA) recently invited me to talk to them about a campaign they wanted to develop which would provide health education to people with HIV. There seems to be some paradox in the HEA educating people with HIV how to be healthy when the HEA is educating those same people through its latest advertising campaign that "the only difference between HIV and AIDS is time".

I want to put things this way, not to embarrass the Chief Medical Officer or the HEA (although I have some exasperation with inconsistent information), but because it shows how, when you have HIV, uncertainty about matters of life and death may be encompassed in a routine telephone call.

The first challenge faced by everyone with HIV is how to live with uncertainty. If one is well, the uncertainty is when and where the first symptom of AIDS will appear. Until yesterday, there was the additional uncertainty of whether the first symptom of AIDS would appear, but the HEA has relieved us of that uncertainty. If one is ill, the uncertainty now is how long you've got and how you will die.

For two people with HIV living together — I live with someone who has HIV, we are both well — it's the uncertainty of not knowing who will become ill first and, if you are lovers, the fear that you may not be able to cope with your lover's illness and death. With that comes the fear that you will have to face your own illness and death already bereaved, alone, in pain and perhaps losing your sanity.

For a single mother with HIV, it's the uncertainty of not knowing when she will have to say goodbye to her child and who will care for it when she has gone. If the child too has HIV, that mother may have to watch her child die, and then prepare to die herself.

Everyone with HIV or AIDS fears the uncertainty of how other people will react. Will they be fearful? Hostile? Judgemental? Blaming? According to the British Market Research Bureau monitoring survey of public attitudes to AIDS during the June 1988 HEA campaign, there was a 45 per cent chance that if you told someone that you had AIDS, their reaction would be, "You've only got yourself to blame."

Many people with HIV prefer not to risk the uncertainty of others' reactions, and put up barriers between themselves and others —

their parents for example — to conceal the fact that they have HIV and to conceal what it is doing to them emotionally, spiritually and physically. Those barriers undermine relationships which may previously have been built on honesty and trust.

This isolation, whether self-imposed, or imposed by others, is increased by the fear that your lover, if you have one, will leave you; or, if you don't have a lover, the fear that no one will want to make love to you ever again. Sexual intercourse is, for many people, the most important means of affirming and maintaining a loving relationship. If you have HIV it may seem as though you can offer so little sexually, safely, that no one will want you and that you will become a very lonely person indeed. You may feel, as I did, that you have become a sexual cripple.

It's the uncertainty of not knowing how long you will be able to keep your job, not knowing how long you will be able to support yourself, keep your home, keep your place in the community, keep your self-respect. It is the uncertainty of not knowing whether, when you become dependent, those who you become dependent on will have the training, the resources, the experience and the skills for you to feel safe in their hands.

Above all, perhaps, it is uncertainty that surrounds loss, whether real or anticipated: loss of an assured future (or at least the assumption of longevity which most of us need in order to set ourselves goals and give ourselves the hope of achieving them); the loss of health, friends, lovers, relationships; the loss of job, income, home and comfort; the loss of security, self-respect and dignity; the loss of love and now, it seems, almost inevitably the loss of life, with perhaps the loss of sanity along the way.

Astonishingly, people with HIV cope with all this: and it seems to me, having worked in the field of AIDS for four years now, that of all the challenges posed by HIV — to medicine, to health care, to social security — the personal, individual challenge of having and living with this disease is the one that is met with most courage, most dignity and most success.

Perhaps this is because people with HIV live in such an uncertain environment that they come to the realization that certainties have to be found within oneself. But all of us who work in the field of AIDS, in whatever capacity, have to live in that uncertain environment and make an individual response to HIV and AIDS within it.

Even the certainties that we do have are, to many people, not credible. For example, I was talking recently to a lecturer who had just given a talk about HIV to an audience of nurses. They all knew you couldn't "catch" HIV by swimming in the same pool as someone with AIDS. "Right," said the lecturer to his audience, "you've gone to the local pool for a swim and there are fifty people with AIDS in the pool. How many of you would jump in?" Not one nurse raised their hand.

We are uncertain about public attitudes to HIV. Those lay beliefs about disease: that it spreads like a miasma through the air (or water), that it is somehow lurking in the environment waiting to pounce, that it is a product of late twentieth-century life or social and moral non-conformity, that it is distributed according to some metaphysical arrangement of justice — these beliefs are extremely deep-rooted and continue to affect public opinion on what should be done about HIV. Ultimately, it is public opinion that determines and constrains the politicians who decide what measures and resources are appropriate in response to HIV.

The problem is compounded by uncertainty about the incidence of the disease. That uncertainty generates a time-wasting and exhausting factionalism, where those responsible for ensuring that the level of resources allocated is proportional to the scale of the problem are caught between accusations by one faction that the threat to the nation's health has been grossly over-stated, and warnings by another faction that HIV is so serious a problem that the health service will collapse under the demands it will create.

An example of the damage this factionalism can do: I serve on a committee formulating national policies for a sector of statutory service provision; the effectiveness and credibility of this committee is in danger of being undermined because the need for these policies is not perceived at local level in some areas and because some people believe it is being manipulated by the "gay lobby".

We lack certainties, and because of that we lack a consensus, and without a consensus there is mistrust and conflict.

The individual challenge for nurses is to overcome their irrational fears; the challenge for doctors is to learn how to care instead of cure; the challenge for the politician is to recognize that his or her political life will probably be shorter than the life of AIDS and to resist the temptation to take short-term "popular" measures which may satisfy public demand for action in response to HIV but which may not serve the longer-term interests of public health.

The government, as one of the subscribers to the London Declaration on AIDS Prevention, acknowledged that discrimination against people with HIV is a threat to public health and promised in January 1988 to: "forge, through information and education and social leadership, a spirit of social tolerance." Some indicators of public attitudes show that while public sympathy for people with AIDS is increasing, tolerance towards gay men has decreased. The government has introduced legislation which colludes with and fuels this intolerance.

I haven't seen any indicators of public attitudes to drug users, but it seems as though the language used to describe them in the context of HIV for example, "a bridging group carrying HIV into the general population" — will help ensure that they are blamed and vilified as the incidence of HIV among heterosexuals increases. We are all challenged to ensure that we don't allow the concepts we use to analyse the epidemiology of HIV — concepts such as "bridging groups" — to engender the threat of social violence against those already threatened by a brutal and violent disease.

I'd like to end on an uplifting note. I believe myself to be extremely fortunate. I belong to a community which has faced, collectively and individually, the social challenges presented by HIV. In that community, people with HIV have not been ostracized; they have not had their autonomy threatened by calls from the uninfected majority for coercive measures to protect them. Members of that community have volunteered in their thousands to provide financial, practical and emotional support to those infected. Members of that community have changed their sexual behaviour in a way that makes it unnecessary to discriminate, even and especially in the act of making love, between those who are infected and those who are not. That seems to me to be a remarkable social achievement. And, as a result, I, and many other people with HIV, have been able to achieve our own personal and private victories against this disease.

I think it is the responsibility of us all, individually and collectively, to ensure that the opportunity to achieve those private victories is made available to everyone over the next few years, whatever the uncertainties.

This is the text of a talk given at a National AIDS Trust conference on "AIDS — Can We Care Enough," held on 1 December 1988, World AIDS Day.

MICHAEL BRONSKI

DEATH AND THE EROTIC IMAGINATION

Now I want you to do something for me. Take me out to Cyprus Hill in my car. And we will hear the dead people talk. They do talk there. They chatter together like birds on Cyprus Hill. But what they say is one word. And that word is "live". They say, "live, live, live, live, live!" It's what they've learned there. It's the only advice they can give. "Just live." Simple! — A very simple instruction.

Tennessee Williams, *Orpheus Descending*

Sex and death are the two most taboo topics in American culture. Few resources or encouragements exist to deal with either in honest or helpful ways. Yet while both are covered in secrecy or denial, sex and death are relegated to distinctly different social positions. Sex, once unmentionable, is now the basis for endless consumer products and marketing devices. Death, on the other hand, is shunted to the bottom of the agenda; avoided until it can be avoided no more. It is the dirty little secret that calls up euphemisms and embarrassed looks. Death doesn't sell anything, or make us feel better, or even bring up all those "good" guilt feelings that add the zest to sex. Death is always something that happens to other people. We have even invented the categories of "natural" and "unnatural" death not so much to classify the types of death but to explain it to ourselves; to draw lines as to why it will not happen to us. On some level everyone knows that death is inevitable, but few people are eager, or equipped, to deal with the fact.

The gay and lesbian liberation movement is very young. Women and men who were thirty during the Stonewall Riots (and many were much younger) are just now over forty-five. It is no surprise then that gay men are having trouble dealing with the huge number of AIDS deaths. The young are never prepared to begin dealing with death — and certainly not the amount of death that has struck the gay male community over the past few years. As of the beginning of 1989 there have been over forty thousand deaths due to AIDS in the US — approximately thirty thousand of those have been gay men.

There is a spectre haunting gay life . . .

Death in this culture has been treated as a personal matter, a family matter. The biological unit pulls closer together, protected by its community, most often centred around a church, and finds ways to deal with the loss. Gay men have also done this. Often gay extended families are stronger, tighter, than nuclear families because they are chosen and built upon mutual support and respect. But these choices and supports do not come easily. In a world that hates homosexuals these are momentous acts whose strength lies in their resilience to the myriad pressures against them.

There is very little — and in some cases *no* —legal or psychological support from outside the gay community to help deal with those issues. There are no secure legal rights for homosexual lovers, often no visiting rights for gay friends. By defining "gay" as purely a sexual activity, and a wrong and sinful one at that, the heterosexual world has not allowed itself to see any social, familial or nurturing aspects of the gay community in its dealings with death. This should not come as any surprise — nor does it for a gay person — since there is no basic respect for the gay world in which the person with AIDS has lived his life.

It is impossible to be a gay male today and not think of AIDS all the time. Not only are you faced with AIDS every time you read a paper, watch TV, or pick up a magazine — it is there over the morning coffee and just before you go to bed at night — but AIDS is on your mind every time the telephone rings, every time a letter from a slightly distant friend arrives. In Boston, a city not very hard hit by the epidemic, I know of thirty men who have died or been diagnosed. People who live in New York or San Francisco may know as many as fifty men who have died or who have AIDS.

The Disappeared

Because the gay male community is large and loosely knit — made up of groups of friends as well as large socializing networks at bars and baths — a great many people know one another casually or just by sight. It has become commonplace over the last five years to presume that a bar regular may be dying or dead if he is absent for a while. The friendship networks are informal enough for one not to know who to ask about a missing man. Often the news of a friend's diagnosis is simply too hard to talk about in the bars or baths he used to frequent. Sometimes life feels like living under a fascist regime as people just disappear without a word.

Since Stonewall, the gay and lesbian community has established a complex and varied network of newspapers and magazines. But the US gay press has not done all that well in helping the community deal with this deluge of death. Coverage of the epidemic has been erratic. While the *New York Native* has gone all out in its medical coverage, too often it is presented in an alarmist, non-informative manner, not very useful to readers who are dealing with their own personal hysterias. On the other hand, *Gay Community News*, which has done some good work about public policy issues, rarely covers medical news. On the more personal level both papers print obituaries of somewhat prominent people — those who may have been known by some segments of the gay community. While this personalizes the effect of AIDS in a tangible manner, it also diminishes the number of cases that come to public attention. This type of obituary also implies, however unintentionally, that some cases are sadder because the men were well known, or because they made some contribution to the gay community while they were alive. This is a comfort to many readers who feel that these few isolated cases — not even the tip of the iceberg — portend no warning to their own lives. The most extreme case is, of course, Rock Hudson, who, while he never came out, even on his death bed, still garnered publicity and sympathy simply for being famous.

Obits: The Lies Between the Lines

Other papers, like the *Bay Area Reporter* in San Francisco, run anything from ten to thirty obituaries every week of regular, everyday gay men who have died of AIDS. This is a chilling sight, especially since many people first see the paper in bars and other gay establishments where it is given away. Reading *BAR* is like walking through a graveyard, or viewing the Vietnam Veterans' Memorial Wall — the only difference is that you knew these people and may have seen them only a week ago. The ultimate effect is to bring the war home; there is no way for a gay man to look at those pages of postage-sized, black-framed portraits and not have some presentiment that this could have been him. And might be in several months time.

Of course the straight press is still worse. The *New York Times* will infrequently acknowledge an AIDS related death as such, but only if the family, or friends, of the deceased makes no attempt to suppress the fact. Or, in a homophobic reversal of this, the media uses AIDS as the final blow in a series of attacks on the dead person, as the *Times* did in the obituary of Roy Cohn. But even when AIDS isn't mentioned, figuring out who is gay and who died of the syndrome is easy: he was thirty-six, a church organist and died after a short illness, leaving parents and a brother in Connecticut; he was forty-two, a respected clothing designer, died after a long illness, leaving a mother and two sisters in Ohio. But these are just the more prominent; the semi-famous by the *New York Times* standards. There is no mention of the thirty-seven-year-old underwriter for an insurance company who died after being hospitalized for eight months, leaving no family because they have not spoken to him since he moved from upstate New York eighteen years ago after telling them he was gay. Nor was AIDS cited in the extensive obituaries of a Boston Latino community leader who died of respiratory complications at the age of thirty-five last spring. Every time one of these obituaries appears, it is not only AIDS that is rendered invisible, but the existence of all gay people.

A startling sense of déja vu occurs for gay men and lesbians when they read these obituaries. It is not unlike twenty years ago when you read gossip columns and newspaper items to see who was married and who was not, to discover who might be gay and who might (with good reason) be hiding their sexuality. You read these things in an attempt to get a sense of community, to find others who were like you, to feel less invisible and alone. The social embarrassment and denial of gay sexuality in the 1950s and 1960s is being re-enacted now in both the gay and straight worlds with the embarrassment and denial of death and AIDS.

Death and the Territory: Movements and Martyrs

The gay community's dealing with death did not begin with AIDS. Before the advent of AIDS the deaths of young gay men I knew were from queer-bashing. Gay men and lesbians knew that transgressing heterosexual limits could be dangerous. In both rural and urban areas, even the most sophisticated, open cities, a gay man or lesbian can be spotted as a homosexual and queer-bashed. And not just beaten but murdered. In the summer of 1986 there were six known gay murders and countless queer-bashings in Boston alone. (And remember not even the most flagrant heterosexuals are beaten just because they are heterosexuals.) For many the connections between death and being gay are very clear. If you were "obvious," if you were "known," if you were seen leaving a gay bar you could be beaten and killed. Death, as it were, came with the territory.

But in some way this ever-present death was, while hard to deal with, clear in its origins. Death was one more form of oppression that occurred because of homophobia — or in less euphemistic terms — because people hated queers. These deaths were part of the social reality that spawned the gay and lesbian liberation movements. Lesbians and gay men learned to deal with these deaths by taking their cues from other, more established social activist movements. On the one hand the dead were seen as martyrs to the "cause". This is clear in the case of Charlie Howard — an effeminate gay man who was murdered by street thugs in Bangor, Maine: there are yearly memorials to him and both legal reform and educational organizing are done in his name. This is not all that different from leftists and labour organizers using the names and images of Joe Hill, Frank Little and Wesley Everest as well as the victims of the Triangle Shirtwaist Factory fire and those killed in the Ludlow massacre and the Haymarket riot hangings. The two most famous quotes in activist folklore are Joe Hill's "Don't mourn, organize," and *Mother Jones*'s "Pray for the dead, but fight like hell for the living." Although the latter makes a nod at acknowledging the dead, both place the emphasis on more immediate political action. These were clearly responses to a cultural inclination to sentimentality (based, in part, on a strain of Christianity) which attempted to secure the status quo by keeping people's minds off the present, and on the past. In the real world, tending to the after effects, the psychological aftershock of death came second to organizing and preparing for the future. The left has not been able to deal with AIDS, in part due to its homophobia, but also because it has always made death a class issue. The left understands death as the result of class divisions which, for example, cause certain people to be drafted to fight in Vietnam, and not others; which deny health care and proper social services to certain groups, and place them at risk in the workplace. But AIDS cuts across class lines, as well as political lines (it is hard for some to come up with any sympathy for Roy Cohn, yet he is as much a victim of AIDS as anyone else).

Sex and the Politics of Death

Since AIDS has become recognized as a problem affecting gay men, the community has done an amazing job of mobilization. There are health crisis centres, AIDS action committees, support systems and direct service groups all over the country. Such organizing has been set up almost entirely by gay men, and to a lesser degree lesbians, with very little help — until recently — from the heterosexual world. To see what gay men have done in such a short period of time is staggering. But what has been done is in the tradition of most work in the gay movement — a direct response to an oppressive situation. Gay men were literally dying in the streets and they were taken in. Gay men were being evicted from their homes, fired from their jobs, denied basic health rights: all of these problems were faced head on.

But the gay movement has only just begun to deal with the psychological response to AIDS and to death. We have not been faced with this much death — this close to home — ever before. In the gay community, both men and women are beginning to realize that there is no more business as usual. The more profound, lasting and deep repercussions of AIDS are just beginning to be felt. They will not become really evident for another few years and will last for years and years after that. Every day that we do not deal with our feelings and reality we will have to do so threefold in the future. In many ways the gay community has followed two of the most traditional responses to death: terror and pity.

The first is the phobic response, a reaction to fear and terror. Some gay men have avoided sex, avoided bars, avoided dealing with their basic sexual identity. Equating gay life with AIDS, and hence with death, they have turned their backs on it. They are filled with fear and loathing for their past lives and their current sexual desires. Not a surprising reaction, since this is the lesson that every homosexual has been taught since birth. Sometimes it takes very extreme forms such as deciding to be heterosexual and to marry, removing one's self from the gay world completely. At other times a more moderate form of denial occurs, such as joining Sex Addicts Anonymous in an attempt to get "dangerous behaviour" under control. But what is even more common is a self-conscious self removal from the active gay world: stopping going out to bars, cutting down the amount of energy put into socializing, sometimes even avoiding the gay press because it is "too depressing". All of these reactions are understandable. AIDS *is* too difficult to think about. But each of these responses is not only an avoidance of AIDS — it is also a denial and a whittling away at the gay community; a slow process that — unless we can find a way to combat it — may have a lasting, disastrous effect on the community itself.

The second traditional response — pity — appears in the guise of sentimentality. You see this attitude in all those articles in major magazines about people with AIDS: "it is such a shame they are dying because they had such great careers, such wonderful lives, such beautiful apartments, such well developed bodies." There is nothing facetious here. Almost every piece on people with AIDS that appeared in pre-1987 *Life, Time, Look* and *Newsweek* was certain to mention their tasteful, well-decorated apartments. Compare these articles to the news and features on people of colour and AIDS, which show their tenement, slum surroundings as the perfect accompaniment — not ironic juxtaposition — to their disease.

Many gay men have had a positive response to this form of mainstream journalism. Looking for the sympathy vote is an easy trap for gay men to fall into because it seems to address oppression: "you may have hated us but now since we are dying you have to like us." Such thinking, of course, is false consciousness because people who hate queers are probably *glad* we are dying — and will take the opportunity to blame us for "spreading" it to the straights. Such thinking adds to the notion that AIDS is a gay disease and reinforces the idea that it is a metaphor for gay life itself.

This whole tradition fits neatly into an old, ingrained, Western cultural tradition, the *Camille* syndrome: the romance of the outlaw, the misunderstood one who may die, but who dies beautifully and with a great deal of pathos and sentiment. Here is the ultimate incurable romantic.

Anyone who has seen a person die of AIDS knows that this disease is not romantic. There are tubes and respirators, open sores and lesions, inflated and cooled mattresses to keep the fevers down to a manageable 103 degrees, balding due to chemotherapy, infections that coat the mouth and make it impossible to eat. Men who were once 200 pounds lie in bed reduced to 110-pound skeletons. Faces once brimming with life and lust are reduced to courageous death masks animated only with the desire to live.

Because of AIDS the gay community is now going to have to begin dealing with death in a manner that speaks to both the mind and the spirit: to social actions and emotions. The effects of AIDS are going to be measured not only in the number of deaths but also in the psychological and emotional ravages on the community; in the feelings of rage, impotence, unresolved emotions and outright terror visited on gay men. The questions raised by this reality range from the obvious, "How do you deal with this amount of personal, communal and political loss?" to the more pressing, and for many more paramount, "How do you have sex when everyone around you is dying?"

The first step in this is to bring death out into the open, not to avoid talking about it and hiding it as though death was a dirty little secret. There is nothing romantic, nothing sentimental — not even anything *more* than usually frightening —about dying of AIDS. It is not, as Susan Sontag might point out, a metaphor for anything. It is like all death: a painful, hard end to the painful and sometimes hard act of living.

The Politics and Death of Sex

Between sex and death gay people have dealt very well with sexual pleasure. We have liberated sex from the confines of the state and religion, from the proscriptions of gender and have legitimized unadulterated sexual pleasure — purely creative, not pro-creative — as an end unto itself. As gay people, we now have to learn to deal with death in the way that we have learned to deal with sex, to see it for what it is and to view it realistically. And along with this we have to try to understand its effect on us, and to acknowledge the place of grief and mourning in our lives.

Up until now the gay movement has learned — partly from the left and partly from our own organizing — to radicalize death: to use death as an impetus for social change. The deaths of Joe Hill, Charlie Howard and also everyone with AIDS have been an incentive to move

forward and to change society. What we are faced with doing now —
in the wake of so much death, so much inconsolation — is to
politicize death; to bring it into our whole lives and to understand
all of its implications for us, both social and personal; to make
death part of a seamless web of existence; neither avoided or
sentimentalized.

We have already learned to politicize sex, to bring sexual desire
into our full lives and to weld the personal and the political together.
From the second wave of feminism (as well as from gay male writers
from Oscar Wilde to Tennessee Williams) we have learned to see
the connections between sex and politics. But there is also a strong
link — a physical one if you believe in the usually acknowledged
routes of HIV transmission —between sex and death. We have to face
that connection. If we are to face it without fear, we must radicalize
sex as we did death; sift through the cultural mythologies and
trappings we attach to sexuality, and try to reimagine it. Education
around AIDS will help create this vision, but we also have to look in
ourselves and understand what sex means to us — and what we
have allowed it to mean in this homophobic culture.

One of the main differences between AIDS organizing and other
political organizing is that many of the people who are doing the
ground work are at high risk — some at very high risk — from the
disease. There is no need — as they used to say — to bring the war
home: it is here already. It is here in the number of AIDS deaths, in
the untold (and continually uncounted) numbers of suicides, and
in the emotional deaths many gay men are suffering.

The gay movement can learn to deal with death in the same way it
has learned to deal with sex: not as a means to an end, as a metaphor,
but as a physical experience, a material, not a moral reality. There is
no inherent mystery surrounding sex and death — those myths are
purely social inventions to control behaviour and make us conform
to certain mores and standards. Sex and death are part of life and the
metaphors, the allegories, the fears and the fallacies that have been
built up around them were invented to keep us from enjoying life
and facing death without fear.

The Bible tells us that the wages of sin are death. But the reality is
that everyone dies regardless of sin. Our traditions tell us that death
is payment for transgressions. As long as we believe somewhere that
sex leads to death it will be impossible to view AIDS without
moralizing and mystifying it.

In the past year there have been some moves to deal with the grief, the loss, the incalculable hurt that AIDS has caused the gay community. The Names Project Quilt — which is now travelling around the country — seems to be not only a concrete memorial but a way for all of us to acknowledge and deal with our own pain, as well as a call to action.

No one, except, perhaps, those who choose suicide, wants to die and certainly no one wants to die of AIDS. We as gay people must learn to face the reality of death with the same energy and imagination we have put into claiming and enjoying our sexual desires and experiences. If we do not deal with death it will continue to cause us more stress, more hurt and more self-doubt. It will be used as another weapon against us — used to deny us ourselves. If death — like sex — remains taboo, clouded behind moralism, abstractions, sentimentality, fear and inadequate notions of politics, we will not be able to claim it as another aspect of our openly gay lives.

Many thanks to Cindy Patton and Charley Shirley for talking through many of the ideas in this article which is reprinted from *Radical America*, vol. 21, nos 2–3 May 1988.

NOTES ON CONTRIBUTORS

Keith Alcorn is an editor of the lesbian and gay cultural quarterly *Square Peg* and works for the National AIDS Helpline. He has curated two lesbian and gay film and video programmes for the Institute of Contemporary Arts in London.

Michael Bronski has been active in gay politics for almost twenty years. He is the author of *Culture Clash: The Making of Gay Sensibility* (Boston, MA 1984). He has written for *Gay Community News, The Boston Globe, Fag Rag, The Boston Herald* and *The Boston Phoenix.*

Erica Carter is the editor of *New Formations.* She was director of talks at the ICA, London, from 1986–88.

Richard Goldstein is a senior editor at the *Village Voice* where he has specialized in rock music, new left politics, the industrialization of fine art and lately, television. He coordinates and writes much of the paper's gay and AIDS coverage.

Jonathan Grimshaw is a co-founder of Body Politic, the oldest British organization for people with HIV. He is an active member of several other AIDS service organizations.

Jan Zita Grover is senior medical editor of an AIDS textbook at San Francisco General Hospital. She taught "Media(ted) AIDS", a course on the cultural politics of AIDS, at the California Institute of the Arts in

1987, and curated "AIDS: The Artists' Response", an exhibition of AIDS related artwork and activism for Ohio State University in 1988. She has published extensively on AIDS in the US and UK.

Meurig Horton is a member of the health education group at the Terrence Higgins Trust and a former consultant to the AIDS division of the Health Education Authority.

Cindy Patton is the Manager of Community Education at the AIDS Action Committee in Boston, of which she was a founding member. She is completing a book on the impact of the US far right on public policy. She is the author of *Sex and Germs: The Politics of AIDS* (Boston, MA 1985), and winner of the American Library Association Gay Book Award, and co-author with Janis Kelly of *Making It: A Woman's Guide to Sex in the Age of AIDS*, New York 1987.

Lynne Segal teaches psychology at Middlesex Polytechnic. Her latest book, *Is the Future Female?*, was published by Virago Press in 1987. She is currently working on a book on men and sexual politics, "Slow Motion: Watching Men, Changing Men", to be published by Virago Press.

Tom Stoddard is executive director of Lambda legal defence and education fund. He is Adjunct Associate Professor of Law at New York University, and a member of the Citizens' Commission on AIDS for New York and northern New Jersey.

Simon Watney is a volunteer at the Terrence Higgins Trust, where he chairs the health education and policy groups. He has lectured and published extensively on many aspects of AIDS, in Britain, Europe and North America, and is the author of *Policing Desire: Pornography, AIDS and the Media*. He is a member of the editorial board of *Screen* and is currently researching a history of the social aspects of the British AIDS epidemic, provisionally entitled "AIDS Britannia".

Jeffrey Weeks currently works in academic administration in London and is a Visiting Fellow at the University of Southampton. He is the author of *Coming Out* (Quartet 1987), *Sex, Politics and Society* (Longman 1981; 2nd ed. 1989), *Sexuality and its Discontents* (RKP 1985) and *Sexuality* (Tavistock 1986).

Tony Whitehead is a founder member of the Terrence Higgins Trust, and a director of Frontliners.

Judith Williamson is a London-based writer and critic. The author of *Decoding Advertisements* and *Consuming Passions*, she teaches film at Middlesex Polytechnic and also works freelance in film and television.

RESOURCES

Publications

In *The Search for the Virus: The Scientific Discovery of AIDS and the Search for a Cure* (Penguin 1988) Steve Connor and Sharon Kingman have written a very accessible yet detailed account of the biomedical history of the epidemic, which does not shirk social and political analysis, albeit in the form of a detective story, in which the role of HIV as the single, all-determining "explanation" of AIDS is assumed all along. None the less, their book conveniently summarizes masses of otherwise scattered information, and provides a thorough international overview of HIV and AIDS around the world. This international perspective is shared and enlarged by two books published by the Panos Institute, based in London, Paris, and Washington. In *Blaming Others: Prejudice, Race and Worldwide AIDS* (Panos 1988), Renée Sabatier has written and edited a valuable survey of the effects of AIDS on people of colour, concentrating on what Dr Jonathan Mann of the World Health Organization has described as the "Third Epidemic" — that of blame. AIDS is repeatedly described as a "misery-seeking missile" in a way that suggests a consciously calculating syndrome, but none the less *Blaming Others* sets out the disproportionate impact of HIV on the black and Hispanic population of the USA, and elsewhere, in a helpful and very timely manner. It is unfortunate that her information about HIV among gay men appears to derive exclusively from Randy Shilts, whose work exemplifies an insidious racism. Also from Panos, *AIDS and the Third World* (1988) offers much information from those countries most severely affected by the epidemic. Cindy

Patton's *Sex and Germs: The Politics of AIDS* (South End Press 1985)
was an astonishingly prescient early response to the complex social
issues raised by the epidemic, and remains an indispensible text,
together with Dennis Altman's *AIDS and the New Puritanism*
(London 1986). The most reliable and accessible current information to the US situation is *The Essential AIDS Fact Book*, edited by
Paul Douglas and Laura Pinsky, New York 1988.

AIDS: Social Representations, Social Practices, (Falmer Press
1989), edited by Peter Aggleton, Graham Hart and Peter Davies,
contains a wide variety of articles on the social aspects of HIV. It also
contains a number of useful articles on the subject of injecting drug
users. Another important collection of articles, focused on the
experience of HIV in the USA is *AIDS: Cultural Analysis Cultural
Activism*, edited by Douglas Crimp (MIT, Cambridge, Mass. 1988).
This is particularly strong on the emergence of AIDS activist
organizations such as ACT UP. At a slight tangent, Anne Karpf's
Doctoring the Media: The Reporting of Health and Medicine (RKP
1988) provides an extremely useful account of the ways in which
definitions and images of sickness and health have been dealt with
in British mass media since the 1920s. The wider field of health
education is also admirably approached via *Concepts of Health,
Illness and Disease : A Comparative Perspective*, edited by Caroline
Currer and Margaret Stacey (Berg 1986). Simon Watney's *Policing
Desire: Pornography, AIDS and the Media* (Methuen 1987) remains
the only extended critique of the cultural and ideological impact of
the epidemic, concentrating on British press and television
coverage. Stuart Hall's *The Hard Road to Renewal : Thatcherism
and the Crisis of the Left*, (Verso 1988) sets out very clearly the
nature of the terrain in which contemporary British cultural politics
operate, with an admirable attention to health care provision as a
central site for political and ideological struggle. We may wish to
read his insights in the larger context of *AIDS and Human Rights :
An International Perspective* (Danish Centre of Human Rights,
Copenhagen 1988) edited by Martin Breum and Aart Hendriks,
which compares HIV related discrimination in countries as far apart
as Britain, the Soviet Union, Sweden, and the USA, with exemplary
thoroughness and analysis.

Periodicals

In Britain, Sharon Kingman edits a regular weekly AIDS information section in *New Scientist*. Tony Whitehead has for several years been producing his magnificent weekly column, "Body Matters," in *Capital Gay*, which is available on subscription from 38 Mount Pleasant, London WC1X 0AP. The "Simon Watney Column" in *Gay Times* also provides a regular in-depth monthly update on HIV related issues. This is available on subscription from 283 Camden High Street, London NW1 7BX. *Body Positive* publishes a useful regular newsletter for people with HIV from PO Box 493, London W14 0TF. But by far the most extensive source of information concerning all aspects of the British epidemic, which also includes overseas listings, is the *National AIDS Manual*, which is published on a subscription basis with regular updates by NAM Publications Ltd., PO Box 99, London SW2 1EL. From the United States, *Focus* has long been an invaluable resource, summarizing debates on medical issues, drug treatments, counselling, and so on. It is published monthly by the University of California San Franciso AIDS Health Project, Box 0884, San Francisco, CA 94143–6430, USA. The most useful information about experimental drug trials and treatments comes from the USA. Three crucial resources are the regular *AIDS/HIV Experimental Treatment Directory*, published by the American Foundation for AIDS Research (AMFAR), 1515 Broadway, 36th Floor, New York, NY 10036, USA; *AIDS Treatment News*, published bi-weekly by John S. James, on subscription from PO Box 411256, San Francisco CA 94141, USA; and *Treatment Issues*, available from GMHC Department of Medical Information, 132 West 24th Street, Box 274, New York NY 10011, USA. Finally, *Project Inform* has played a major role in disseminating AIDS information, and their regular publications can be obtained from 347 Dolores Street, Suite 301, San Francisco, CA 94110, USA.

Organizations

Most parts of Britain are now covered by a wide variety of AIDS service organizations, both voluntary and run by local authorities. Information about all of these may be obtained from the National AIDS Manual, or from The Terrence Higgins Trust, 52–54 Gray's Inn Road, London WC1X 8JU (Helpline: 01 242 1010). Frontliners, the leading national organization for people with AIDS, can be contacted by writing to BM AIDS, London WC1N 3XX (tel: 01 831 0330). Body Positive, the original group for people with HIV, can be reached via PO Box 493, London W14 0TF (tel: 01 373 9124). Positively Women, a group for women with HIV or AIDS, can be contacted via Soho Hospital, Soho Square, London W1, or telephoned direct (01 734 1794). The Black Communities AIDS Team (BCAT) is at 47A Tulse Hill, London SW2 2TN (tel: 01 671 7611/2). The Terrence Higgins Trust Helplines are open from 3 pm to 10 pm every day (01 242 1010), and the free National AIDS Helpline is open twenty-four hours daily (0800 567123).